I'm a Loser

A Go-To Book for All Dieters

I'm a Loser

A Go-To Book for All Dieters

Diane Brown

Printed in the United States of America

First Printing, 2018

ISBN 978-1-947656-72-7

ISBN10: 1947656724

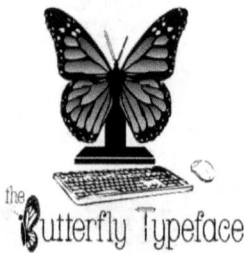

the
Butterfly Typeface

The Butterfly Typeface Publishing
PO BOX 56193
Little Rock AR 72215

www.thebutterflytypeface.com

Disclaimer

"I'm A Loser" is designed to provide information about the subject matter covered. This book is not a replacement for medical   services and should not be used to assist with diagnosis or treatment. The publisher and author are not engaged in rendering professional medical services through the use of this literature. If medical assistance is required, the services of a competent and qualified professional should be sought.

The information provided should not be considered as all-inclusive. Therefore, this text should be used only as an example and entertainment, not as the ultimate source of medical information. Furthermore, this book contains information on medical information and techniques only up to the printing date.

The purpose of this book is to educate and to entertain. The author and   Butterfly Typeface Publishing shall have neither liability nor responsibility to any person or entity with respect to any loss or damage caused or alleged to be caused directly or indirectly by the information contained in this book.

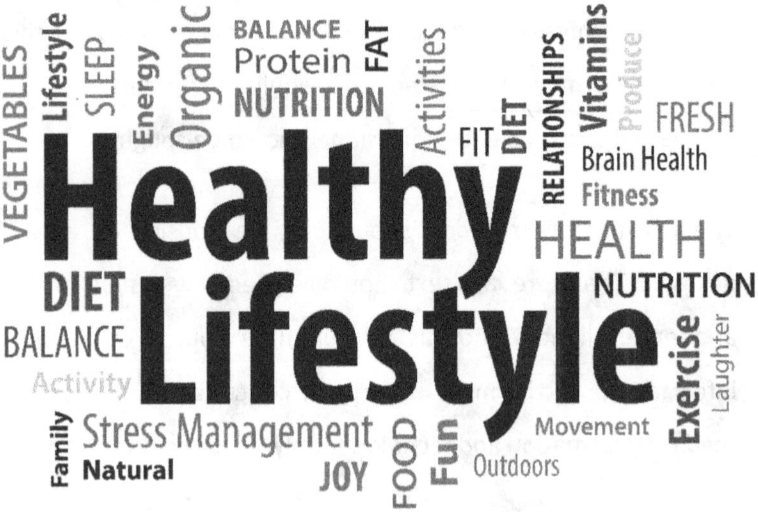
VEGETABLES
Lifestyle
SLEEP
Energy
Organic
BALANCE
Protein
NUTRITION
FAT
Activities
FIT
DIET
RELATIONSHIPS
Vitamins
Produce
FRESH
Brain Health
Fitness
Healthy
HEALTH
NUTRITION
DIET
BALANCE
Activity
Lifestyle
Exercise
Laughter
Movement
Family
Stress Management
Natural
JOY
FOOD
Fun
Outdoors

If you desire to lose or prevent weight gain,
THIS BOOK IS FOR YOU!

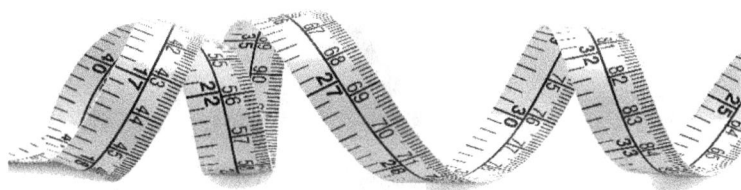

Alert!

An increasing number of physicians are eager to cooperate with patients who want to improve their diets, health, and lifestyle. If you are under medical care, taking medication, or about to embark on a radical diet change, make an appointment to see your doctor for a physical and consult with him about your health plans.

Table of Contents

Acknowledgments

To my family and friends who provided your success
stories and exceptional support, please know, that you are
the "key" ingredient in this book.

Thank you, DB

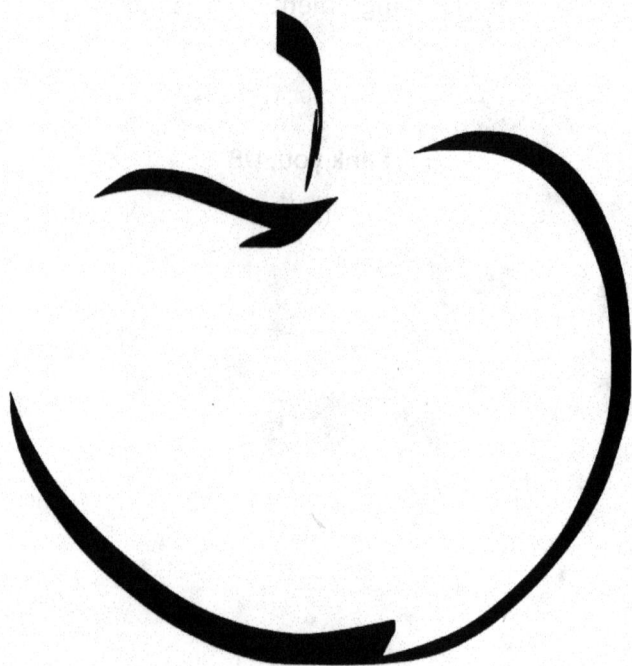

Dear Reader,

Your choosing to purchase this book, tells me that you too are a "Lifetime Loser." You will forever seek a healthier lifestyle. You will all, as losers, continue this journey. There will be rocky trenches along the way, hills, and even mountains. There will be days you will want to give up, "and yes" you will give "in" but you will never "give up" because you are a lifetime loser. I welcome you! I'm excited about the journey you are about to embark. I encourage you to simply take it "one day at a time" Feel my energy throughout every conversation of this book. Let's enjoy this life journey!" Choose "good over bad," and love yourself enough to get back up every time!

Author, Diane Brown

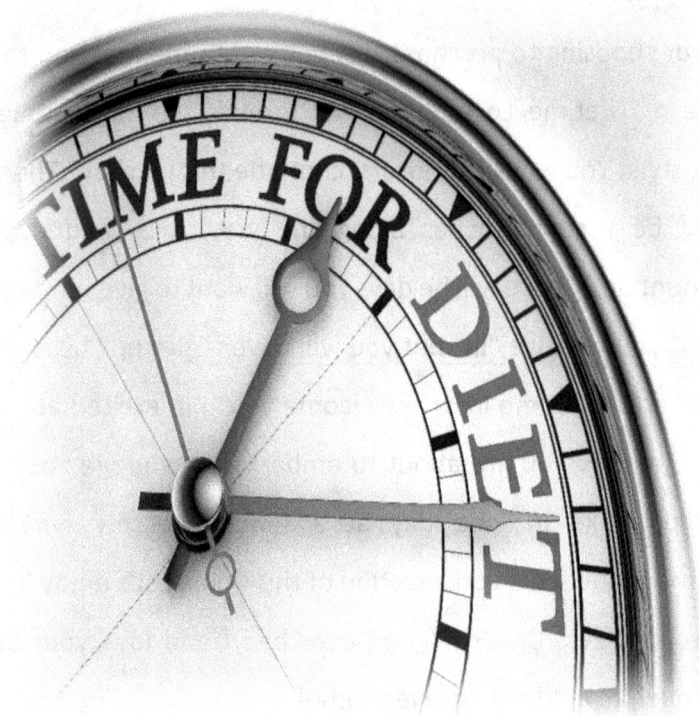

Introduction

The good news is that weight gain can be prevented! By choosing a lifestyle that includes good eating habits and daily physical activity. By avoiding weight gain, you avoid higher risks of many chronic diseases. *All listed in this book.* If your goal is to prevent weight gain, then you'll want to choose foods that supply you with the appropriate number of calories to maintain your weight. In addition to a healthy eating plan, an active lifestyle will help you manage your weight.

By choosing to add more physical activity to your day, you'll increase the number of calories your body burns. This makes it more likely you'll maintain your weight. Although physical activity is an integral part of weight management, it's also a vital part of health in general. Regular physical activity can reduce your risk for many chronic diseases, and it can help keep your body healthy and strong.[1]

Chapter One: Reasons for Weight Gain

I suppose we all have our thoughts and clichés of why we gain weight. Well, first of all, we eat too much and work out too little, but who would have "thunk," *gravity*, yes, *gravity* would cause so much turmoil. Below I've listed some studies regarding possible reasons for weight gain.

Effects of Gravity on the Body
(Read more @ www.evolutionhealth.com)

You can't see, touch, taste, or smell it, yet you can feel its effects every day and experience its cumulative damage on our bodies over a lifetime. No other force affects us so dramatically. Have you ever noticed that your pants felt a little tighter around the waist at the end of the day? Did you realize that after the age of 20, you've been losing an average of ½ in height every 20 years? Do you suffer from varicose veins, swollen feet, or an aching back? If you responded yes to any of these questions, you are a victim of the inescapable force of gravity. Your organs become compressed. Your waist measurement increases. You probably call these, "love handles;" we call them "compression wrinkles" because they are, in part, a direct result of compression of the spine.

Thyroid (Hypothyroidism) and Weight Gain
(Read more @ www.webmd.com)

When the amount of thyroid hormone your body makes goes down, the number on your scale sometimes goes up. Your thyroid glands send hormones into the bloodstream that help keep your metabolism in check. When you don't make enough of these hormones, that process slows down. That puts the brakes on body functions. You might feel cold, tired, or sluggish. Your body might also hang onto salt and water. That causes bloating.

Menopause and Weight Gain
(www.bodylogicmd /"Weight Gain in Men")

Maintaining proper weight is a challenge for people of all ages. However, the older you get, the more difficult it can be. It has been found that 90% of women experience weight gain between the ages of 35 and 55, not coincidentally, during perimenopause and *menopause*. While nutrition, exercise, and lifestyle are critical elements to weight loss, balancing your hormones after the imbalance that menopause caused, is vital to your success in maintaining a healthier weight. Hormones and weight gain are closely related. If your hormones are not balanced, you can gain weight especially with too much cortisol or too little progesterone, testosterone, or estrogen. <u>Bioidentical hormone therapy</u> may tip the scales in your favor.

While the cause and effect relationship is not clear, it is apparent that there is a strong connection between weight gain in men and andropause related hormonal imbalances. Low testosterone and high cortisol seem to increase body fat, especially in the midsection, and decrease muscle mass in men. This body fat appears to further the hormonal imbalance by converting testosterone into estrogen. Male weight gain coupled with muscle loss means more weight to carry and less muscle to carry it with resulting in fatigue and low energy levels.

Reasons For Weight Gain
(www.prevention.com)

Here are seven health issues that could be standing between you and your ideal weight:

1. *Depression-* Many anti-depressant medications cause weight gain. If you are not medicating, there's evidence that feelings of depression can correlate to weight gain.

2. *You're taking the wrong Rx-* There's a long list of medications that can cause weight gain: birth control pills, excess hormones for hormone therapy, steroids, beta-blockers for heart disease, blood pressure, anti-seizure meds, breast cancer medications, and even some migraine and heartburn medications.

3. *Your gut is slow-* Digestive issues, including slow bowel movements, may also account for excess pounds.

4. *Your body's missing certain nutrients-* Being *low in magnesium, iron, or having a vitamin* D deficiency can compromise your immune system, zap your

energy levels, or alter your metabolism in ways that make it harder to take healthy-lifestyle steps.

5. *You're getting older-* It's the one condition that's unavoidable. We don't burn as many calories at 40 or 50 as we did at 20, so we need more exercise and less food to keep our metabolism going. Some studies show that exercise might be even more important than the diet for long-term weight maintenance.

6. *You have plantar fasciitis (foot condition)-* Many musculoskeletal conditions, including plantar fasciitis, but also osteoarthritis and knee or hip pain can result in unintentional weight gain. Plantar fasciitis certainly can cause you to cut back on your activity enough to cause weight gain.

7. *You have Cushing's Syndrome-* Weight gain accompanied by high blood pressure, osteoporosis, and changes in your skin tone and quality, including purple or silvery stretch marks on your abdomen and ruddy cheeks, could be sign that your body isn't processing nutrients the way it should due to a cortisol-producing tumor on one of your adrenal glands. One of the revealing signs of Cushing's

syndrome is how fat is distributed. The distribution appears primarily in the mid-section of the body, leaving the arms and legs to look more slender.

A Few Solutions
(www.prevention.com)

Constipation: If constipation is your symptom, trying probiotics can help your digestive tract work properly. Staying hydrated is critical, along with a diet chocked full of fiber-rich foods!

Wrong medication: If you suspect your medication is affecting your waistline, your doctor may be able to find an alternative treatment that won't have that particular side effect.

Your body is missing certain nutrients (Vitamin D): It's nearly impossible to consume enough milk or to get enough sunlight to compensate for low Vitamin D. It's important to know that it could take a while to find your right dose of Vitamin D. If you take too much, you can get kidney stones. You need to have your blood tested every 3 months, so your doctor can make adjustments to your dose.

Getting Older (50's club): Eating lean proteins will help your body to burn calories more efficiently. Carbs are something your body tends to burn more slowly and even store in your body more readily. Choosing low-fat proteins, reducing carbs, and exercising at least 4 days a week, are good ways to help avoid unnecessary pounds.

Feet (plantar fasciitis) or other limb pains: Modify your exercise program; swap biking or swimming in place of weight-bearing exercise. Seek out a physical therapist who can design an appropriate plan for your specific needs.

Depression: Many anti-depressant medications cause weight gain. If you're not taking pills, there's evidence that feelings of depression can correlate to weight gain. "If I see patients who are taking anti-depressants and that could be the culprit of their weight gain, I may wean them slowly off of the drug," says Dominique Fradin-Read, MD, MPH, an assistant clinical professor at the Loma Linda School of Medicine in California. "I may then put them on Wellbutrin (Always check with your doctor!) instead, which actually helps with weight loss." If your meds are not the blame, seek out some workout buddies or a support group. All are a great way to increase social support, which can help depression.

Chapter Two: Benefits of Exercise

(PREVENTIONS: 1994 *Lose Weight Guidebook*)

Every system of your body works better if you stay fit. The person who gets enough exercise is less likely to die of heart disease, even if he or she is overweight, smokes have high blood pressure or high cholesterol, or a family history of heart problems. People who get enough exercise are less likely to die of cancer than those who don't. The standard recommendation for minimum fitness is three walks a week, 20-30 min per walk. This activity level should bring major health benefits to the previously sedentary person.

Regular physical activity can improve your muscle, strength, and boost your endurance. Exercise delivers oxygen and nutrients to your tissues and helps your cardiovascular system work more efficiently. When your heart and lung health improve, you have more energy to tackle daily chores. Beginners, as well as more advanced fitness levels, will see the most significant benefits if they work out three to four times a week. The main thing is that you schedule a *rest day* between the different sessions. You should take at least one day off after two consecutive days of strength training.

What Can Exercise Do for You?

Exercise improves your mood and reduces depression, stress, and anxiety. It gives you more energy and helps keep you focused. It also combats many health conditions and diseases, promotes better sleep, and enables you to relax. It slows the aging process and makes your older years more enjoyable. Exercise strengthens and boosts your immune system, improves confidence, and body image. It sharpens your memory and helps with learning. Exercise improves your sex life by increasing your blood flow. It helps control addictions to tobacco, alcohol, and other drugs and improves digestion and eases constipation.

Cardiovascular Health

Cardiovascular exercise forces the heart to work harder in order to supply working muscles with adequate blood and oxygen. Over time this strengthens the heart muscle. This allows us to be more active during the day without being fatigued.

CARDIO WORKOUTS

Step Aerobics, Brisk Walking, Elliptical Trainers, Running, Biking, Jumping Rope, Swimming

Weight Management

Exercise is a great tool for managing weight by increasing the number of calories used throughout the day. Exercise can help manage any type of weight-bearing exercise (walking, jogging, biking, strength training) which place stress on the skeletal system. Bones adapt to that stress by increasing their production of *osteoblast*, which is responsible for bone remodeling and growth. Weight-bearing exercise can be a great way to delay and possibly improve bone loss (osteoporosis).

Lower Cholesterol

HDL is the good cholesterol that helps to remove **LDL** (bad cholesterol) from the bloodstream as waste. By doing cardiovascular exercise, we can increase the amount of circulating **HDL**, which can help improve the blood lipid profile and work to decrease **LDL** levels, which are mostly determined from genetics and **"Food Choices."**

Blood Pressure

High blood pressure can be a sign of stress, cardiovascular disease, or other health issues. Regular physical activity helps to ward off high blood pressure by maintaining clean arteries, a healthy heart, and circulatory function. Exercise also reduces stress, which helps decrease blood pressure as well.

Sleep

According to the National Sleep Foundation's 2013 Sleep in America poll, more than three-fourths of exercisers (76-83 percent) say their sleep quality was very good or fairly good in the past 2 weeks, compared to only 56% of non-exercisers. This shows the correlation between exercise and sleep quality.

Anti-Aging

Exercise is physical stress applied to the body. There are two types of exercise stress that play a role in reducing the effects of aging:

1)Mechanical stress (resistance training)

2)Metabolic stress (cardio)

High-intensity exercise can provide mechanical or metabolic stress necessary to stimulate the production of naturally occurring anabolic steroids, which promote muscle protein synthesis and increase lean muscle mass. Both help to mitigate the effects of the aging process. Exercise floods the brain with BDNF (brain-derived neurotrophic factor), a substance that boosts brain cell growth and strengthens cell-to-cell connections, which works to increase cognitive function.

Stress

Exercise helps to lower blood pressure, which can be a marker of high stress. Exercise releases serotonin and dopamine; the "feel good" neurotransmitters, which make you feel happier, more relaxed, and less stressed.

Job Performance

The increase in BDNF in the brain due to exercise makes brain cells stronger, healthier, better connected, and larger, which leads to increased learning capability. Exercise balances neurotransmitters and other chemicals in the brain. These substances influence brain activity related to mood, attention, learning, motivation, and arousal. That's why you're likely to feel calmer, more alert, and more focused after exercise.

Chapter Three: Obesity-Related Health Conditions

"Every time you eat or drink, you are either feeding diseases or fighting it."

There are many diseases and health issues associated with obesity. They include the following:

*High blood pressure, *Type2 diabetes, *Coronary heart disease, *Stroke, *Gallbladder disease, *Osteoarthritis, *Sleep Apnea and breathing problems, *Some cancers (endometrial, breast, colon, kidney, gallbladder, and liver,) *Low quality of life, *Mental illness such as clinical depression, anxiety, and other mental disorders, *Body pain and difficulty with physical functioning.

Let's discuss a few of these and the effects that bad eating has on them:

TYPE 2 DIABETES
(www.webmd.com)

While not everyone with Type 2 diabetes is overweight, obesity and lack of physical activity are two of the most common causes of this form of diabetes. The good news is Type2 can be managed! What you *eat* makes a big difference, when you have diabetes.

There or 4 key things diabetics must focus on:

1. **Carbs-** Some carbs are simple like "sugar" other carbs are complex like those found in beans, nuts vegetables, and whole grains. Yes, *Complex carbs are better for you!*

2. **Fiber-** Fruits, vegetables, whole grains, nuts, beans, and legumes help with digestion and blood sugar control.

3. **Fat-** Diabetes makes you more likely to get *heart disease,* so you will want to limit unhealthy fat such as saturated fat and trans fats.

4. **Salt-** Diabetes raises your risk of getting high blood pressure. Too much salt can add to that risk. Your physician may suggest that you limit or avoid salt intake.

10 FOODS TO REDUCE BLOOD SUGAR LEVELS

(Sweethealthblog.blogspot.com)

This article presents ten foods that prevent and lower the sugar levels in the blood. By consuming these superfoods on a regular basis, you can stabilize and even reduce the blood sugar levels. It is also important to mention that patients who already take diabetes medications should pay attention to their diet choices because what they eat, and drink can significantly affect the way their organs manage the disease.

1. **Cinnamon**- Cinnamon contains components that have the ability to promote glucose metabolism and reduce high levels of bad cholesterol. Recent scientific study showed that only ½ a tsp. of cinnamon powder per a day significantly decreases fasting blood glucose levels and increases insulin sensitivity in patients who suffer from diabetes.

2. **Sweet Potatoes**- Sweet potatoes contain the beta-carotene antioxidants, but also are high in Vitamin A, Vitamin C, potassium, and fiber. All these

ingredients were proven to be helpful in controlling the blood sugar. However, it is important to mention diabetic patients should not consume regular potatoes because they have a higher glycemic index alternative than sweet potatoes. You can prepare grilled or baked, yet it is advised to prepare potato with the skin on.

3. **Beans-** Beans are high in dietary fiber, protein, magnesium, and potassium. These minerals are essential for patients who suffer from diabetes. Studies show that beans slow down the process of digestion and thus help maintain blood sugar after eating a meal. You can choose between pinto, navy, white, lime, chickpea, soybeans, or back beans.

4. **Dark Green Leafy Vegetables-** Dark green leafy vegetables are one of the healthiest foods because they are high in Vitamin C, soluble fiber, magnesium, lots of calcium, and are very low in calories and carbohydrates.

5. **Berries-** Berries of all kinds (strawberries, blueberries, cranberries, etc.) are a rich source of antioxidants, vitamins, and fiber which are

extremely helpful in controlling the blood sugar levels.

6. **Fish**- It is a well-known fact that fish is a rich source of omega-3 fatty acids and one of the healthiest meals. Doctors explain that in order to get all of the benefits, we should eat fish at least twice a week. For diabetic patients, cold water fatty fish, such as salmon, sardines, halibut, herring, mackerel, and tuna are the best choice.

7. **Whole Grains**- Magnesium, chromium, omega-3 fatty acids, and folic acid are some of the wide variety of nutrients contained in whole grain foods. Scientist explains that the whole grains have the ability to lower the blood sugar level and also effectively reduce your blood pressure and LDL (bad cholesterol).

8. **Nuts**- Walnuts are abundant in healthy fats, vitamins, fiber, and a lot of minerals including magnesium and Vitamin E, which have the ability to stabilize the blood glucose levels. Other nuts are pecans, almonds, and peanuts.

9. **Olive oil**- If you are looking for a healthy oil for cooking, olive oil is the best choice. The antioxidants

and monounsaturated fats contained in olive oil significantly reduce the risk of heart diseases and in same time reduce the insulin resistance. In order to get all of the benefits of the olive oil, always choose extra virgin olive oil.

10. **Yogurt**- Yogurt is high in protein, Vitamin D and calcium. There are many scientific studies which have shown that participants who consume a lot of calcium-rich foods lose weight more easily. Calcium-rich foods also reduce the chances of insulin resistance.

Note: Besides healthy foods, it is also important to exercise regularly and try to maintain healthy body weight.

SLEEP APNEA
(WebMD)

"In adults, the most common cause of obstructive **sleep apnea** is excess weight and obesity."

The treatment involves the following:

Reach and maintain a healthy weight, humidify your bedroom, adjust your sleeping position, avoid excessive alcohol, smoking, and overuse of sedatives.

OBESITY AND CANCER
(www.cancercenter.com)

The *Lancet Oncology* researchers attributed 500,000 new cancer cases worldwide in just 1 year to *obesity*. Carrying too much weight is already a known risk factor for certain cancers, including breast, colorectal, and pancreatic. But the findings suggest obesity may play an even greater role.

OBESITY AND GALLBLADDER DISEASE
(www.health247.com)

If you're overweight or obese, your risk for gallbladder disease (typically an inflamed or infected gallbladder with gallstones) is higher. Since gallstones are made of cholesterol, if you have high cholesterol, it can add to your risk of getting gallstones and feeling the discomfort that comes with them.

OBESITY AND OSTEOARTHRITIS (OA)
(www.healthline.com)

Obesity is one of several factors that can contribute to *OA*, and age is another big factor. The older you get, the more wear and tear you put on your joints. Losing extra weight helps remove pressure on your joints. These activities can help lower your risk of developing *OA* or at least cause a reduction in symptoms.

OBESITY AND BODY PAIN
(www.spine-health.com)

While it has not been thoroughly studied how excess weight can cause or contribute to back pain, it is known that people who are overweight are often at greater risk for back pain, joint pain, and muscle strain than those who are not obese.

OBESITY AND HEART CONDITIONS
(www.drugs.com/mcd/heart-attack.com)

A heart attack occurs when the flow of blood to the heart is blocked, most often by a build-up of fat, cholesterol, and other substances, which form a plaque in the arteries that feed the heart (coronary arteries). The interrupted blood flow can damage or destroy part of the heart muscle.

A heart attack, also called a myocardial infarction, can be fatal, but treatment has improved dramatically over the years. It's crucial to call 911 or emergency medical help if you think you might be having a heart attack.

OBESITY AND STROKE
(www.slideshare.net)

High blood pressure, high cholesterol, and smoking are major risk factors for a *stroke*. Those affected have a higher incidence of the risk factors of a *stroke*. Obesity/Overweight are primary risk factors for stroke for men and women of all races.

Stroke Warning Signs:

- Sudden numbness or weakness of the face, arm or leg, especially on one side of the body.
- Sudden confusion, trouble speaking or understanding.
- Sudden trouble seeing in one or both eyes.
- Sudden trouble walking, dizziness, loss of balance or coordination.
- Sudden, severe headache with no known cause.

(Ref: American Stroke Association)

Heart Attack Warning Signs:

- Chest discomfort (uncomfortable pressure)
- Pain in one or both arms, back neck, jaw, or stomach. Shortness of breath, this may occur with or without chest discomfort
- Other signs, cold sweat, nausea, or lightheadedness.

(Ref: American Heart Association)

Chapter Four: Feed Thy Spirit

(Devotions for Dieters)

"God's bread of life is nonfattening."

Let's face it: dieting wouldn't be as hard if the food didn't taste so good. Like anything good, we want to get as much of it as we can. It's easy to place a high value on the food we eat. But there is such a thing as too much of a good thing. God has given us many freedoms, but one we should not abuse is the freedom to consume as much food as we want. No one can limit what we eat except ourselves.

We need to realize that our daily bread supplies what we need, not what we want. Excessive eating is selfishness, and selfishness is a sin. When we feel the urge to overeat, let us turn to God and nourish ourselves on the true bread that comes from Him, His Word.

"This is that bread which came down from heaven: not as your fathers did eat manna, and are dead: he that eateth of this bread shall live forever." John 6:58

The stomach is a spoiled brat! When we miss even one meal, it kicks up a fuss and makes us feel as though we're going to starve. Of course, we're in no danger whatsoever, but once our stomachs get started, it is hard to ignore them. To diet means to engage in mind over matter. We need to realize that we can get by on a lot less food than we actually eat. We need to renew our minds, change our thinking, and decide that we're not going to be made a slave to our stomachs. When we refuse to be ruled by anything but the Spirit of God, then we truly please Him.

"And be not conformed to this world: but be ye transformed by the renewing of your mind, that ye may prove what is that good, and acceptable, and perfect, will of God."
Romans 12:2 (KJV)
"Sit out the urge it will pass"
(freedomnotfear.tumblr.com)

And if I asked you to name all the things that you love, how long would it take for you to name "yourself?"

Dieting involves a constant struggle between two intense desires: The desire to lose weight and the desire to indulge in the foods we love. This is not an easy struggle. We are double minded. God wants all of his children to learn to be single-minded. Once we decide that something is important, we should learn to stick to it. That's not as easy to do on our own. For that reason, it is helpful for us to draw close to God. He will listen as we tell our troubles. The closer we are to God, the more He can help us through difficult times. If we ask Him to, God will help us become single-minded. He is as anxious as we are to see us attain our goal.

"...For the righteous Lord
loveth righteousness:
his countenance doth behold the upright..."
"Dieting is no reason for self-pity."

Long-distance runners train themselves to think of the finish line. They visualize it just ahead. They say this keeps them from wanting to give up somewhere along the way.

The reward of crossing the finish line is worth more than any pain or discomfort along the way...Dieters can learn from this. Instead of dwelling on how hungry we are or how much we long for fatty foods, we should continually think in terms of the rewards that await us at the end. Christians follow Christ with the hope of a Heavenly reward. Faith means we await something yet to come. Dieting means we live in the hope of trimming down and looking fit.

"...the reward of our diet
is greater than the sacrifice..."
"He that followeth after righteousness
and mercy findeth life,
righteousness and honour."
Prov. 21:21

Warfare Prayers

By the blood of Jesus, I speak confusion to the camp of my "ENEMIES!" I lift up the powerful blood of Jesus against all evil spirits fighting against me. I sprinkle the blood of Jesus upon all my properties. Let the blood of Jesus cleanse my bloodline of all inherited "CURSES!" Let the blood of Jesus soak and dissolve all the "MOUNTAINS" before me, in Jesus name. Let every evil mark on me be washed and sanitized by the blood of Jesus!

—warfare prayers

A Prayer To Lose Weight

Guide me, Lord, as I strive to lose weight, You are my light and my anchor, and with You, I know all things are possible. Help me this day to make healthy choices and give me the strength to fight against destructive cravings that negatively affect my health. You said, "The Lord upholdeth all that fall, and raiseth up all those that be bowed down." As I bow before you today, raise me up; help me towards my goals. I have been taught that anything that replaces God is an idol. Help me to reject any unhealthy habit in which I seek false comfort. For You are my one true comfort and salvation. In Your name, I pray, Amen.

I REBUKE

Cancel & destroy every assignment and attack of the enemy and cancel every curse and negative word ever spoken over my life
in the powerful name of *JESUS CHRIST!*...
AMEN, AMEN, & AMEN!

STAND STRONG

May you stand strong in the face of enemy threats. May you remain confident even if an army rises up against you. May you put your flag in the ground and declare that if God is for you, who can stand against you? Far greater is *HE* who is in the world. May you rise up this day and walk forward in holy confidence and humble dependence. You are God's beloved, and He will guard and guide you, shelter and provide for you, and bless and establish you. Jesus loves you, and nothing and no one can change His mind about you. He's sold on the idea of you! May you live like you're His because you are! A blessed and beautiful day to you!

I SAID A PRAYER

I said a prayer for you today, and I know God must have heard. I felt the answer in my heart, although He spoke no word! I didn't ask for wealth or fame (I knew you wouldn't mind). I asked Him to send treasures of a far more lasting kind! I asked that He'd be near you, at the start of each new day to grant you *health* and blessings, and friends to share your way! I asked for happiness for you, in all things great and small, but it was for His loving care, I prayed most of all! (Printed in Italy)

THANK YOU, LORD

Dear God, Thank you. When I turned on my kitchen tap this morning, clean water came out. When I opened my pantry door at lunch, I couldn't decide what to eat because I had too many choices. When my family and I sat down at the kitchen table for dinner and held hands to say grace, I felt the warmth of their healthy hands and their happy hearts, and as I laid in bed reading stories to my little babes, we all looked up to appreciate the roof over our heads... You have blessed my life tremendously. I'm sorry I don't say thank You enough. Forgive me. Amen.

(Redcarpetlife.me)

Healthy Eating Go-To Scriptures
(www.lysaterkeurst.com)

God has given me power over my food choices.

I'm supposed to consume food. Food isn't supposed to consume me. 2 Cor. 12:9-11, "but he said to me, my grace is sufficient for you, for my power is made perfect in weakness...for when I am weak, then I am strong."

I was made for more than to be stuck in a vicious cycle of defeat.

Deut. 2:3, "You have circled this mountain long enough. Now turn North."

When I am considering a compromise, I will think past this moment and ask myself, "How will I feel about this choice tomorrow morning?"

1 Cor. 6:19, "Do you not know that your body is a temple of the Holy Spirit, who is in you, whom you have received from God? You are not your own. You were bought with a price. Therefore, honor God with your body."

When tempted, I either remove the temptation or remove myself from the situation:

Rom. 6:19-20, "I put this in human terms because you are weak in your natural selves. Just as you used to offer the parts of your body in slavery to impurity and to ever-increasing wickedness, so now offer them in slavery to righteousness leading to holiness."

When there's a special event, I can find other ways to celebrate rather than blowing my healthy eating plan...

Rev. 3:8, "See, I have placed before you an open door that no one can shut."

I have these boundaries in place, not for restriction but rather to define the parameters of my freedom.

1 Cor. 10:12-14, "So, if you think you are standing firm, be careful that you don't fall! No temptation has seized you except what is common to man. And God is faithful; he will not let you be tempted, he will provide a way out so that you can stand up under it. Therefore, my dear friends...flee..."

OLIVE LEAF TEA

God's remedy was written in the Bible. This powerful recipe is 3500-years-old! The olive leaf has been used for ages for nourishment and medicine. *The Bible* shares many instances of the olive tree. The olive leaf was used even before Christ.

Ezekiel 47:12,
"The fruit thereof shall be for meat and the leaf thereof for medicine."

Olive leaves are cultivated since ancient times and are used as food and medicine around the world. What most people do not know is that olive leaves have the greatest healing properties, and may help in recovery from pneumonia, gonorrhea, tuberculosis, influenza, meningitis, hepatitis B, herpes, and many others thanks to the most important compound, *Oleuropein* ("search" it's amazing benefits).

Tea made of olive leaves will help in the fight against various diseases but will also strengthen the immune system and provide you extra energy. This tea should be consumed after chemotherapy or when you are stressed and want to relax.

Olive Leaf Tea (Recipe)

Ingredients

- 15-20 dried olive leaves
- 2-3dl (deciliter measurement) US convert- 3dl = 1.2 cups of boiling water

Collect the leaves in the spring and leave them to dry in the air. When dry, put them in a glass jar, and store in a cool, shaded place.

Directions

Put the leaves in the 1.2c of boiling water and cook them for 10min. Take them off and let the tea cool for 15min. Add honey or lemon, if you prefer. This tea is excellent for overall health and should be consumed several weeks in a row to attain its benefits.

(http://holisticplanet24.com/gods-remedy-written-in-the-bible-this-powerful-recipe-3500-years-old-cure-all-diseases/ OR wwwhealthtipsportal.com)

SCRIPTURE CAKE

A scripture cake, also known as Bible Cake or Old Testament Cake, is one of those cake recipes that has been around for many, many years. The recipe is written entirely by using the scriptures from the Bible. To be able to bake one, you needed to know your Bible scriptures. It was especially popular in the 1830s-50s, with ladies and young girls. For young girls, it was used to teach them to cook and their Bible verses at the same time. For the ladies of the house, it was an opportunity to show off their cooking prowess and their knowledge of the Bible.

Scripture Cake (Recipe)

Ingredients

- 1 c Judges 5:25
- 1 c Jeremiah 6:20
- 1 tbsp 1Samuel 30:12
- 3 Jeremiah 17:11
- 1 c 1 Samuel 30:12
- 1 c Nahum 3:12
- 1/4 c Numbers 17:8
- 2 c 1 Kings 4:22
- 2 Chronicles 9:9
- a pinch of Leviticus 2:13
- 1 tsp Amos 4:5
- 3 tbsp Judges 4:19

Directions

Preheat oven to 325 degrees, cream the first 3 ingredients. Beat in 3 Jeremiahs until light, adding one at a time. Add the next three ingredients and beat once more. Sift together Kings, 2 Chronicles, Leviticus, and Amos. Add 2 mixtures together and blend well. Add milk and blend. Pour into a well-greased loaf pan and bake for 1 ½ hrs. or until well done.

INTERPRETATION

Ingredients

- 1 c butter
- 1 c sugar
- 1tsp honey
- 3 eggs
- 1 c raisins
- 1 c chopped figs
- ¼ c chopped almonds
- 2 c flour
- spices, such as cinnamon, allspice, nutmeg, a pinch of salt. 1tsp leavened-baking soda or baking powder
- 3tbsp milk

Directions

Preheat oven to 325 degrees. Cream together the first 3 ingredients. Beat in 3 eggs until light, one at a time. Add the next 3 ingredients and continue to beat. Sift together, flour, spices, salt, and baking soda or baking powder. Add the two mixtures together and blend well. Blend in milk. Spray pan with spray oil. Pour batter into bundt or loaf pan and bake for 1 ½ hrs or until done.

(Source: "scripture cake recipes")

Note: This, of course, is not the "healthiest" cake recipe, but you can tweak some of the ingredients. Instead of 1c butter replace ½ the amount of butter with "applesauce." Even better, if you don't mind a denser, more moist cake, you may use all applesauce! Instead of 1c sugar, use 3/4c sugar plus 1tbsp Natural Honey. Instead of 2c white flour, use 2 c oat flour.

UNLEAVENED BREAD
(Cooks.com)

The idea for this recipe came from I Kings 17:10-16, the story of Elijah and the widow.

Ingredients

- 1c whole wheat flour (extra for dusting)
- 2tbsp extra virgin olive oil
- ½ c water

Directions

Combine the ingredients. Then, put dough onto floured surface. Knead for five minutes; roll out until about 1/8in. thick. On either parchment paper or a greased cookie sheet, bake in a pre-heated 350-degree oven for 20 minutes.

Chapter Five: Jump Start Diets

(favpins.com/6-types-of-intermittent-fasting/)

These diets are not offered as long-term weight loss diets. They are merely 'quick results' for weight loss. It is suggested that you go into a healthy lifestyle change diet immediately after completing any 'jump start' diet. (See chapter 6: Best Lifestyle Diets)

Intermittent Fasting

Intermittent Fasting is an eating pattern that determines consecutive eating and fasting time frames. Basically, you don't eat for a particular amount of time during the day or week; then, you fit all your meals into a certain time frame. During your fasting period, you're allowed to drink water, black coffee, *matcha*, and green tea or other natural teas without added sugars.

There are several plans, such as:

1. ***EAT-STOP-EAT*** –Fast once or twice a week for 24hrs. You might have dinner on Tuesday and not eat again

until the same time on Wednesday, after that you just follow your regular diet. This fasting method can bring great results; however, this method may be difficult to stick to if you're new to weight loss.

2. **THE 16:8 DIET** – You fast for 16 hrs. a day and eat during the other 8. 16 hrs. sounds like a lot, but the reality is part of that 16 hrs. is your sleeping hours! For example, you could have dinner at 6pm and not eat anything else until 10am the next day. But you can choose your eating window yourself depending on your preferred dinner or breakfast time or your schedule!

3. **THE 5:2 DIET** – This diet is great for those who find it hard to stick to a certain meal plan. What you do is eat what you usually would 5 days a week and the other two days you only eat about 500-600 calories. Your two fasting days shouldn't be consecutive. It's recommended that you start with this simpler diet if you need to work up to the other methods. (This is my preferred)

On the fast days, choose high protein foods and veggies. Fill your plate with leafy greens, celery, cucumbers, bell peppers, and broccoli. Protein keeps you full for longer; therefore, it should be the main focus of your fasting meals. Good lean sources include steamed fish or chicken, tofu, egg whites, and beans. Protein shakes are ideal on fast days. Drink lots of water and tea to curb hunger. Avoid soft drinks and fruit juices on fast days because they contain empty calories.

If you're hungry drink water with psyllium husk, (this type of fiber forms a gel in your stomach, keeping you full longer). It's recommended that you choose your "fast days" when you are normally your busiest or away from home all day. Soups are low in calories and keep you satisfied on fast days. *MyweightLossDream.co.uk*

By all means, research other listed "Intermittence Diets" as well. Most importantly, consult with your physician before beginning any "Diet Plan."

6 types Of Intermittent Fasting:
(favpins.com)

1)Alternate Day Fasting:

It's the most effective fasting method when it comes to weight loss as it allows you to cut your total calorie intake by up to 50%, while also being able to eat without restriction on the non-fasting days.

2)One day per week fasting:

While this style of fasting doesn't lead to the same weight loss gains as alternate day fasting, it is believed to be a more healthful approach which allows you to cleanse your body without placing it under too much stress.

3)Up to the 9th hr. Fasting:

This style of fasting is great for beginners as it allows you to eat every day but still experience and enjoy the benefits of fasting.

4)One meal per day fasting:

This technique involves eating a single meal each day and fasting for the rest of the day. It's a flexible form of fasting, and the single meal can be eaten at a time that suits you best. It can also be as small or large as you like.

5)Nightly Fasting:

This involves stopping eating a few hrs. before sleeping and extending the body's natural fast that occurs during the night.

6)16/8 Fasting:

This involves fasting for 16 hrs. each day and doing all your eating within an 8 hr. window of your choosing.

7-Day Cabbage Soup Diet (Wonder Soup)
(Divascancook.com)

Drink 8-10 glasses of water daily, eat your cabbage soup as much as you like and lose up to 10 lbs. in 7 days.

DAY1/ Eat only fruit, except bananas.

DAY2/ Start the day with a baked potato, then eat only vegetables, except corn and other starchy vegetables (google starchy vegetables).

DAY3/ Eat only fruits & veggies, except bananas and starchy veggies.

DAY4/ Eat only bananas, milk, and yogurt.

DAY5/ Eat only tomatoes (6-8) and protein (fish, chicken, or turkey).

DAY6/ Eat only protein and non-starchy veggies.

DAY7/ Eat only fruits, vegetables, and juices (no bananas or starchy veggies)

Cabbage Soup Diet Recipe
(Author: Divas Can Cook)

Ingredients

- ½ head of cabbage, chopped
- 1c celery, diced
- 1c white or yellow onion, diced
- 1c carrots diced
- 1 green bell pepper, diced
- 2-3 cloves garlic, minced
- 4 c chicken broth
- 14oz can of basil, oregano, garlic diced tomatoes
- 1tsp oregano
- 1tsp basil
- ½tsp red pepper flakes
- few shakes of black pepper
- ½tsp salt(optional)

Directions

Heat 2tbsp of olive oil in a large pot over med. heat. Add celery, onions. bell peppers, and carrots; sauté until slightly tender. Stir in garlic, pour in chicken broth, and stir in tomatoes and cabbage. Bring to a boil; reduce heat. Cook until cabbage is tender. Stir in oregano, basil, red pepper flakes, black pepper, and salt. Taste broth and adjust seasoning if needed. Serve and enjoy!

Note: This makes enough for about 3 days

48hr.-weight-loss jump start
(Boonsri Dickinson/ Fitnessmagazine)

(Narrator: Dawn Jackson Blatner, an American Dietetic Association spokesperson and FITNESS advisory board member.)

This 2-day weight-loss jump start has a workout and diet plan to help you drop pounds, feel healthier, and full of energy.

(The diet and workout plans are listed on the following pages.)

Day 1 Diet

Breakfast (roughly 300 calories):

Nutty Oatmeal with Apples

Prepare a ½c dry quick oats, w/ ½c original soy milk, 1tbsp walnuts, top w/ 1 small chopped apple.

Google other 300 calorie healthy breakfast choices

Lunch (roughly 400 calories):

Fresh Tomato & Bean Stuffed Pita

1 med. whole wheat pita, ½c canned white beans, 1c chopped tomato, 2tbsp chopped fresh basil, 2tbsp vinaigrette dressing.

Heat the beans, tomatoes, and basil, stuff into Pita, and spice its flavor w/ vinaigrette.

Google other 400 calorie healthy lunch choices

Snack (roughly 100 calories):

½c plain Low-fat Yogurt w/tsp Honey

Dinner (roughly 400 calories):

Salmon w/Quinoa and Broccoli

3oz of grilled salmon, 1c chopped broccoli florets, 1tsp pine nuts, 1 juiced lemon, ¾c quinoa

Enjoy your grilled salmon, flavored w/lemon juice and pine nuts, and steamed broccoli over quinoa

Google Other 400 calorie healthy dinner choices

DAY 1 WORKOUT

For best diet results: Begin by stretching and deep breathing, Do at least 2/ 30min or a 1hr workouts within the day!

Day 2 Diet

Breakfast (roughly 300 calories):

Almond Toast w/Blueberries

2 slices of toasted whole wheat bread, 1tbsp almond butter, 1c fresh blueberries

Spread the Almond butter on the toast, and eat w/side of blueberries

Lunch (roughly 400 calories):

Chopped Spinach Salad

2 cups spinach, 1 large hardboiled egg, 1 medium baked potato, diced, 1c carrots chopped, 2tbsp vinaigrette salad dressing, add the chopped ingredients to spinach and toss with dressing

Snack (roughly 100 calories)

Celery with Sunflower Butter, 1tbsp sunflower butter with two medium celery sticks

Dinner (roughly 400 calories)

Chicken Veg. Stir-Fry w/Brown Rice

Ingredients

- ½c cooked brown rice
- 3oz grilled chicken breast diced
- 1tbsp sliced almonds
- 1tbsp fresh cilantro, chopped
- 1c mixed veg

Directions

Top chicken w/almonds and cilantro. Eat with a side of rice and mixed veg.

DAY 2 WORKOUT

For best results try to get in at least two 30 min. or 1 hr.
workout.

Reminder: This is only a 48-HOUR/2-DAY DIET!

2 DAY SHOPPING LIST

Dry quick oats

Original soymilk

Walnuts

1 small Apple

1 med. Whole Wheat Pita

1 can White beans

Tomatoes

Fresh Basil

Plain low-fat yogurt

Honey

3oz Grilled salmon

Broccoli florets(chopped)

Pine nuts

1 Lemon

Quinoa

Loaf of Whole Wheat bread

Almond butter

Carton of fresh blueberries

1 bag spinach

1 egg

1 med. Baked potato

Carrots

Bottle of vinaigrette salad
dressing

Sunflower butter

2 med. Celery Stalks

1 small bag of Brown rice

3oz Grilled chicken breast

Sliced almonds

Fresh cilantro

1 bag of frozen vegetable
medley

14 Day Lemon Diet
(Fabulousfashionzandstyle.blogspot.ca)

Every morning before breakfast drink lemon juice and water:

Day1   Drink the juice of 1 lemon and 1 cup of water

Day2   Drink the juice of 2 lemons and 2 cups of water

Day3   Drink the juice of 3 lemons and 3 cups of water

Day4   Drink the juice of 4 lemons and 4 cups of water

Day5   Drink the juice of 5 lemons and 5 cups of water

Day6   Drink the juice of 6 lemons and 6 cups of water

Day7   Drink the juice of 3 lemons and 10 cups water; mix with a teaspoon of honey and drink during the whole day

Day8   Drink the juice of 6 lemons and 6 cups of water

Day9   Drink the juice of 5 lemons and 5 cups of water

Day 10   Start reducing the amount of 1 lemon and a glass of water (Do this for days 11 and 12 too)

Day 13   Drink the juice of 1 lemon and 1 cup of water

Day14   Drink the juice of 3 lemons and 10 cups of water; add a teaspoon of honey and drink before breakfast (If possible drink the remainder throughout the day)

Note:

While you drink this lemon juice, try to eat healthier food. In the morning you can eat any kind of oats; for a snack, you can eat some fruit. The lunch should contain proteins, so you can eat meat with vegetables. Try not to eat after 6pm. If you have a desire to eat, make a vegetable salad. Avoid eating fruits in the evening hours.

(Lose 10-20 lbs. in 2 weeks)

3-Day Military Diet
(welldietbase11.info)

The *military diet* is currently one of the world's most popular diets. It is claimed to help you lose weight quickly, up to 10 lbs. in a single week.

DAY 1

BREAKFAST: 1 cup coffee or tea w/caffeine, ½ grapefruit, 1 slice bread wh. Wheat toast,2tbsp peanut butter

Lunch: 1c coffee or tea, w/caff., 1 slice of whole wheat bread or toast, ½c tuna

Dinner: 3 ounces of any meat (size as a deck of cards) 1c green beans, ½ banana, 1 small apple, 1c vanilla ice cream

DAY 2

Breakfast: 1 slice bread or toast, 1 egg prepared as you like, ½ banana,

Lunch: ½ c cottage cheese, 1 boiled egg, 5 saltine crackers,

Dinner: 2 hot dogs (no bun), ½ banana, 1c broccoli, ½c carrots, ½c ice cream

DAY 3

Breakfast: 1 slice of cheddar cheese, 1 small apple, 5 saltine crackers

Lunch: 1 slice of bread or toast, 1 egg prepared as desired.

Dinner: 1c tuna, ½ banana, 1 c vanilla ice cream

Note: For the remaining 4 days of the week, you are encouraged to eat healthily and continue to keep your calorie intake low.

4day-Morning Banana Diet
(Japan's Most Popular Diet for Weight Loss)

Breakfast

Eat Bananas for breakfast (3-4 medium to small size) and drink room temp water.

Note: Very Important! Either drink water 30 min. before meals (even your morning bananas) or 2 hrs. after your meal – NOT while having your meal.

Lunch and Dinner

Eat normally for lunch & dinner. Avoid unhealthy snacks, fried foods, and desserts. If you can't get rid of the sweet tooth, you can have dark chocolate (small square) or 1-2 cookies. It's suggested to eat these at about 3 pm in the afternoon (allows enough time to burn off before bedtime).

Note: For full info about this simple diet plan, search Japanese Morning Banana Diet Review. It mentions this would be a great plan to switch to after the 3-day military diet. The remaining 4 days do the "morning banana diet."

Dukan Diet -10 Pounds In 7 Days
(wwwforkf.com)

Day1 <u>Pure Protein</u>- eat only protein-rich foods, such as lean meat, fish eggs, poultry (10 min. walk)

Day2 <u>Add Vegetable</u>- add veggies to your proteins, this day except for potatoes and beans (15 min. walk)

Day3 <u>Add Fruit</u>- add fruits to your daily meals, except bananas, grapes, and cherries (15 min. walk)

Day4 <u>Add Bread-</u> Spoil yourself with 1-2 slices of whole wheat bread (20 min. walk)

Day5 <u>Add Cheese</u>- you can now eat 1-2 slices of cheese per day (20 min. walk)

Day6 <u>Add Starches-</u> In this last 2 days you are allowed to eat starches, such as potatoes, rice (30 min. walk)

Day7 <u>Celebrate!</u> - Have a small cheat meal to celebrate your weight loss (30 min. walk)

The Boiled Egg Diet
(https://edrugsearch.com/health-benefits-of-eggs/)

There are a number of benefits to point out regarding this simple egg diet. For one, it doesn't require you to buy a lot of products.

Also, this diet has been shown to increase metabolism and decrease the amount of fat in the body, and you get all the health benefits of eggs

However, like most other diets, it's vital that you stay hydrated! You need to drink 8-10 glasses of water each day.

This Boiled Egg Diet can help you lose up to 22 lbs. in 14 Days

WEEK 1:

Monday:

- Breakfast: Start with 2 boiled eggs. Then, eat one whole citrus fruit (your choice).
- Lunch: 2 sweet potatoes and 2 apples
- Dinner: Large chicken tossed in salad, or 1 piece of chicken on the side

TUESDAY:

- Breakfast: 2 boiled eggs, but you can change the citrus fruit.
- Lunch: Dark green vegetables and a chicken salad
- Dinner: Vegetable salad should be paired with 1 orange and 2 boiled eggs.

WEDNESDAY:

- Breakfast: 2 boiled eggs and a citrus fruit
- Lunch: Low-fat cheese paired with 1 tomato and 1 piece of sweet potato.
- Dinner: lettuce salad with 1 piece of chicken

THURSDAY:

- Breakfast: 2 eggs and a citrus fruit
- *LUNCH:* 1 whole fruit (your choice)
- *DINNER:* Salad w/steamed chicken

FRIDAY:

- Breakfast: 2 eggs and a citrus fruit.
- *LUNCH:* Steamed veggies and 2 boiled eggs.
  DINNER: Salad w/grilled fish

SATURDAY:

- Breakfast: 2 boiled eggs and citrus fruit.
- *LUNCH:* 1 Fruit.
- *DINNER:* 1 piece of chicken w/steamed veggies

SUNDAY:

- Breakfast: 2 boiled eggs and citrus fruit.
- *LUNCH:* Salad w/steamed veggies, 1 piece of chicken.
- *DINNER:* Steamed vegetables

WEEK 2:

MONDAY:

- Breakfast: 2 boiled eggs and citrus fruit:
- **LUNCH**: Salad w/small serving of chicken.
- **DINNER:** 1 orange, salad w/2 boiled egg

TUESDAY:

- Breakfast: 2 boiled eggs w/citrus fruit.
- **LUNCH:** 2 boiled eggs w/steamed veg.
- **DINNER:** Salad and grilled fish

WEDNESDAY

- Breakfast: 2 boiled eggs w/citrus fruit.
- **LUNCH:** salad w/piece of chicken.
- **DINNER**: Orange, veg. salad, 2 boiled eggs

THURSDAY

- Breakfast: 2 boiled eggs w/citrus fruit.
- **LUNCH:** Steamed Veg. w/low-fat cheese and 2 boiled eggs.

- **DINNER:** Salad w/chicken

FRIDAY

- Breakfast: 2 boiled eggs w/citrus fruit.
- **LUNCH:** Salad w/salmon or grilled fish.
- **DINNER:** 2 boiled eggs w/salad

SATURDAY

- Breakfast: 2 boiled eggs w/citrus fruit.
- **LUNCH:** Salad w/chicken.
- **DINNER:** Fruit of your choice

SUNDAY

- Breakfast: 2 boiled eggs w/citrus fruit.
- **LUNCH:** Steamed Veg. w/chicken.
- **DINNER:** Same as lunch...

Protein Shake Recipes
(Reddit.com)

Peach Cinnamon- 2 scoops vanilla protein powder, ½ ripe peach, 1c milk, 1 small container of Greek yogurt, 1c spinach or spring greens, ¾c cinnamon toast crunch, 4+cubes of ice.

Banana Nut Muffin Shake- 1 ½ scoops vanilla protein, 1 lg frozen banana, 1tbsp almond butter, 8-16oz water

Very Berry Vanilla- 2 scoops vanilla protein powder, 2c frozen mixed berries, 1tbsp walnuts, ½c low-fat, plain almond milk yogurt, 1c spinach, 1tbsp ground flaxseed, 12oz water.

Mocha Banana Wake-up Call- 1 scoop mocha protein powder, 1 lg frozen banana, 1c chilled coffee, ¼c coconut or almond milk, 2-3tsp coconut oil, 1tsp maca, 4+ cubes of ice.

A glass of Apple Pie- 2 scoops vanilla protein powder, 1 sliced, cored apple, 2tbsp almonds, ¼c uncooked gluten-free oats, a dash of cinnamon, 1c spinach, 12oz water milk or yogurt, 4+cubes of ice.

Chocolate- Peanut Butter-Banana- 2 scoops chocolate protein powder, 1 lg frozen banana, 2tbsp peanut butter, 1c spinach, 1tbsp dark cocoa bits or powder, 12oz water milk or yogurt.

Mango and Tart Cherry- 1 scoop vanilla protein, 1c chopped mango, ½c frozen tart cherries, ½c 100% tart cherry juice, 1c coconut water, 4+cubes of ice.

Pina Colada Power Shake- 2 scoops vanilla protein powder, ½ lg frozen banana, 1c pineapple chunks, 1tbsp ground flax seed, 1c spinach, 2tbsp natural coconut flakes, ½c plain yogurt or almond yogurt, 12oz water, milk or yogurt, 4+ cubes of ice.

Watermelon Breeze- 1 scoop vanilla protein powder, about a ¼ slice of a small watermelon, 4+cubes of ice.

Super Chocolate Mint- 1 scoop chocolate protein powder, ¾c dark chocolate almond milk, 1tbsp walnuts, 2tbsp unsweetened cocoa powder, 1tbsp cacao nibs, 2 mint leaves, ¼c water, 4+cubes of ice.

Key Lime Pie- 1 scoop vanilla protein powder, 1tbsp lime juice, ½c cottage cheese, 1tbsp sugar-free vanilla pudding mix, crushed graham cracker topping, ½c water, 4+cubes of ice.

"Tea for Two" (Herb Teas)
(www.theindianspot.com)

Tea Remedies

Tea for a sore throat (Honey)-1tbsp honey, 1 ½tsp lemon juice, 1c water, a dash of cinnamon.

Tea for sleep (Chamomile) 3-4 dried chamomile flowers or use a chamomile tea bag and 1c boiled water

Tea for bloating (Peppermint tea)1tsp peppermint leaves, 1tsp of fennel seeds, honey (to taste), few drops of lemon, and 1c boiling water. Steep peppermint leaves in hot water for 15 min. along with fennel seeds and strain. Add in a few drops of lemon juice and sweetener.

Tea for clear skin (green tea)1 green tea bag, 1c boiled water. Allow steeping for 15 min.

Tea for Anxiety (Basil) 1 tbsp dried basil, honey (to taste) and 1c boiled water. Allow tea to steep for 30 min.

Tea for a headache (Ginger), 2c water, 1-inch piece of ginger, peeled and sliced into rounds and 1-2 slices lemon (optional)

Chapter Six: Best Lifestyle Diets!

(www.top10weightlossplans.com)

How do you choose a diet that is right for you? Research. Do your research first. Determine your needs and goals, read the instructions and requirements. Finally, what has others said about the diet? Then make your decision.

I've done some research, and I don't mind sharing my results with you!

The 'Best' Diet Categories
(Ref: WebMD)

Best overall: Dash Diet

Best for weight loss: Weight Watcher

Best for Diabetes: Dash Diet

Best for Heart Health: Ornish Diet

Best for healthy eating: Dash Diet

Easiest to follow: Weight Watchers

Best Commercial Plans: Weight Watcher

Best Plant-based: Mediterranean Diet

MAYO Clinic Diet
(Visit Mayo Clinic Diet)

The Mayo Clinic Diet aims to help you lose weight and keep it off. It focuses on identifying bad habits and making positive diet modifications while adding in the right amount of physical activity for every individual.

It features a personalized diet plan, daily advice and support, exercise plans, and more, all for just $5 per week.

This diet features:

1. Tools to break bad habits
2. Customized meal plans
3. Personalized workouts.

(Lose up to 6-10 lbs. in 2 wks.)

Mayo Clinic Diet Testimonials

"In 2 years, I lost 105 lbs. I went from a size 24 to a size 10! My blood sugar went from 101 to 93! I can proudly say that I have completed 2 half marathons!

"I lost 77 lbs. What I immediately liked about the *Mayo C Diet* is that it's really about common sense. It's clear how many servings of each food you should have each day."

Nutrisystem

(www.nutrisystem.com)

NUTRISYSTEM: Lose up to 13 lbs. & 7 inches overall in your first month

Nutrisystems are easy to follow meal plans which have helped millions lose weight and lead healthier lives. Its key to weight loss with its six small meals throughout the day, to leave you satisfied and to keep cravings at bay.

NUTRISYSTEM **TURBO** for **MEN**: You will eat 5 times a day, enjoy fresh fruits and vegetable, and learn to eat healthy on your own with 4 flex meals a week. You can lose an average of 1-2 lbs. per week. Plus, each 4-week plan is delivered right to your door!

NUTRISYSTEM DIABETES PLANS: Lose weight and manage your diabetes the delicious way! It helps promote weight loss and stabilizes blood sugar. It provides balanced nutrition for safe, effective weight loss and has delicious, top-rated frozen foods available *Nutrisystem D plan.*

NUTRISYSTEM VEGETARIAN PLAN: "This plan may be just for you." It's a 4-week vegetarian plan that's easy to follow. Dietitian approved. Choose from over 90 vegetarian selections and unlimited access to counselors and dietitians. It has free online tracking tools and an app as well as free FedEx shipping.

South Beach Diet
(www.southbeachdiet.com)

South Beach Diet Plan: The SBDP has delicious fully prepared meals designed for clean eating and optimal health. This high protein, low-carb plan is made to ***Burn Fat & transform your Metabolism!*** It is a safe and healthy plan for fast weight loss: Phase 1) 7-day body reboot, this phase resets your metabolism for fast weight loss! Phase 2) This is the beginning of steady weight loss! Phase3) "You've got this." Enjoy all foods in moderation! With this easy to follow plan, including fully prepared meals delivered straight to your home, you'll lose weight quickly and learn the way to maintain a healthy weight without hunger or deprivation.

Bistro MD Plan

(www.bistromd.com)

Bistro MD Plan: "We are consistently ranked #1 in diet meal delivery and have been named the *Best Meal Delivery Diet of 2013.*" Each meal is prepared using only the freshest ingredients. Scientifically proven healthy meal delivery plans developed by Dr. Cederquist to target fat.

Lisa- 50 lbs. lighter! Cindy-55 lbs. lighter! Mia- 40 lbs. lighter! Gretchen 15 lbs. lighter! Chris 40lbs lighter! Lisette 32 lbs. lighter! Erin 25 lbs. lighter!

Green Blender Diet Plan

(greenblender.com)

Green Blender Diet Plan: Weight Loss Smoothies Delivered, Green Blender sends everything you need to make farm-fresh smoothies at home. *How it works-* Receive order; open the box. Blend baby blend. Drink and enjoy!

What people are saying:

"I love your service, lost weight while feeling great!"

"I lost 40 lbs. and energy level is so much higher!"

"Losing weight only after 3 weeks, takes the trouble out of shake making!"

Diet To Go
(www.diettogo.com)

<u>Diet To go:</u> From our delicious, healthy and portion-controlled meal plans to our expert support staff and tools, we have over 25 years of experience helping people reach their goals.

Healthy Chef
(site??)

<u>Healthy Chef</u> Creations/healthychefcreations.com: Choose one of their convenient meal programs or do your own healthy meal planning. Customize meals from their A La Carte menu. It's that simple.

Best Diets Overall!
(Julene Stassou. MS RD)

*Dash Diet- prevent and lower higher blood pressure, which is why it's called the *Dietary Approaches to Stop Hypertension.*

*TLC Diet- endorsed by the *American Heart Association* as a heart-healthy regimen that can reduce the risk of cardiovascular disease.

*Weight Watchers- A very popular and effective lifestyle change program.

*HMR Program- **H**ealth **M**anagement **R**esources Program

*Mayo Clinic Diet- Eat well, Enjoy life, Lose weight!

*Jenny Craig- No other weight loss solution offers a dedicated personal consultant together with delicious foods for real results.

*Mediterranean Diet- 28 Day Kickstart Plan for lasting weight loss.

1200 Calorie Diet
(Fitness Quest Eating Plan)

What you eat minus what you burn is the determining factor to weight gain, loss, or maintenance. Are you taking in more calories than you need to fuel your body? Do you know how to calculate the number of calories you need?

Use this formula to find out (fit2print.tumblr.com):

- ✓ 4.35 x your weight in pounds =
- ✓ 4.7 x your age =
- ✓ 4.7 x your height =
- ✓ Add all 3 of those answers above to 655

This number is the number of calories your body needs simply to exist.

Important Note:

1200 CALORIE DIETS ARE GREAT FOR WEIGHT LOSS! MOST HEALTH PROFESSIONALS SUGGEST NEVER TO GO BELOW 1200 CALORIES.

If you are exercising during this 1200 calorie plan, you will need to increase your calories to 1500 (maybe more depending on the intensity of your workout).

Let your increase be more in adding more proteins and or vegetables.

As always, check with your doctor before beginning any diet.

1200 Calorie Menu

DAY 1

BREAKFAST, - 1 plain waffle, 1 tbsp. Maple syrup, 1 tsp butter or margarine, 8 oz water or caffeine-free, non-caloric beverage.

LUNCH- 1 c skim milk, 1 salad with romaine lettuce, ¼ c each carrots, green peppers, cabbage, celery, 1 tsp lite salad dressing, 1 whole grain roll.

AFTERNOON SNACK- ½ c sliced strawberries, 6 oz fat-free flavored yogurt.

DINNER- 3 oz sirloin steak, (lean only, broiled or grilled without added fat). 1 c rice, 1 tsp butter or marg. ½ c cooked carrots, 1 mixed green salad, 2 tbsp. Fat-free dressing.

EVENING SNACK- Orange.

DAY2

BREAKFAST- ½ c oatmeal, cooked w/2 tsp brown sugar, ½ c skimmed milk, 1 c orange juice.

LUNCH- 1oz turkey breast, mustard, or fat-free mayonnaise, 2 slices whole wheat bread, 1 apple.

AFTERNOON SNACK- ½ c skim milk, 1 c strawberries.

DINNER- 2 oz chicken breast (no skin), baked broiled, or grilled. 1 small baked potato, 2 tsp butter or margarine, 1 c green beans, 1 mixed green salad, 2 tsp fat-free dressing.

EVENING SNACK- Low-fat milkshake made with: 1 c skim milk, 1 c fat-free ice-cream.

DAY3

BREAKFAST- 2 pancakes, 4in round, 1 tsp fruit spread or maple syrup.

MORNING SNACK- 1 c skim milk,1 sliced peach.

LUNCH- 1 salad with mixed greens, 1 tsp fat-free dressing, 6 saltine crackers, 3 oz tuna fish, (albacore, water packed), 1 apple.

AFTERNOON SNACK- ½ oz. chocolate (about 4 chocolate kisses)

DINNER- 1 c cooked pasta, ½ c spaghetti sauce (meatless), 1 mixed green salad, 1 tsp fat-free dressing.

EVENING SNACK- 1 c skim milk, 1 whole graham cracker.

DAY4

BREAKFAST- ½ c orange juice, ½ c cereal, 1 c skim milk, 1 c strawberries,

MORNING SNACK- 2 tsp reduced fat peanut butter, 2 rice cakes.

LUNCH- 1 c vegetable soup, 1 mixed green salad, 2 tsp fat-free salad dressing, 1 c skim milk, 6 saltine crackers.

AFTERNOON SNACK- 1 Apple.

DINNER- 1-piece (5 oz) flounder, or other white fish, baked, broiled, or grilled. 1 med. Baked

DAY5

BREAKFAST- ½ English muffin,1 egg poached, ½ grapefruit, 1 c skim milk.

MORNING SNACK- 1 pear.

LUNCH- 2 oz turkey breast or lean ham, ½ large whole grain pita, 2 sliced carrots, 1 c skim milk.

AFTERNOON SNACK- 1 peach.

DINNER- 2 slices cheese pizza, 1 large mixed green salad, 1 tsp fat-free salad dressing.

DAY6

BREAKFAST- 1 bagel, 1 tsp light cream cheese, 1 c orange juice.

MORNING SNACK- 6 oz fat-free, flavored yogurt.

LUNCH- 2 oz lean hamburger, grilled or broiled, 1 tsp ketchup, 1 hamburger bun, ½ tomato, sliced, 1 c skim milk.

DINNER- 1 c angel hair pasta, 2 oz boiled shrimp, 1 tsp olive oil w/garlic on pasta, 1 mixed green salad, 1 t fat-free dressing, ½ c cooked green beans.

DAY7

BREAKFAST- 1 slice French toast, 1 c fresh blueberries, 1 c skim milk.

MORNING SNACK- 1 orange.

LUNCH- ¼ c cottage cheese, 1 mixed green salad, 1 tsp fat-free dressing, 1 whole wheat roll, 1 c skim milk, ½ c sliced carrots.

DINNER- 3 oz baked or broiled cod, 1 c noodles, 2 tsp butter or marg. ½ c applesauce, 1 c mixed vegetables.

EVENING SNACK- ½ c fat-free pudding.

1500 Calorie Menu

DAY1

BREAKFAST- 2 plain waffles, 1 tsp maple syrup, 1 tsp butter or margarine, 8 oz water, or caffeine free, non-caloric beverage, ½ c orange juice.

MORNING SNACK- 1 c skim milk, ½ cinnamon bagel.

LUNCH- Salad with romaine lettuce, ¼ c each carrots, green peppers, cabbage, celery, 1 tsp lite salad dressing, 1 oz turkey breast, 1 whole grain roll.

AFTERNOON SNACK- ½ c sliced strawberries, 6 oz fat-free flavored yogurt, 1 tsp crunchy whole grain cereal.

DINNER- 3 oz sirloin steak, (lean) broiled or grilled, 1 c rice, 1 tsp butter or margarine, ½ c cooked carrots, 1 mixed green salad, 2 tsp fat-free dressing.

EVENING SNACK- 1 Orange.

DAY2

BREAKFAST- 1 c oatmeal cooked, 1 tsp brown sugar, ½ c skim milk, 1 c orange juice.

MORNING SNACK- 1 Apple.

LUNCH- 1 oz turkey, mustard or fat-free mayonnaise, 2 slices whole wheat bread, 1 ½ c sliced cucumbers and carrots, or other raw vegetables.

AFTERNOON SNACK- 1/2 c skim milk, 1 c strawberries.

DINNER- 3 oz skinless chicken breast, baked, broiled, or grilled, 1 med. baked potato, 2 tsp. butter or margarine, 1 c green beans, 1 mixed green salad, 4 tsp regular Italian salad dressing.

EVENING SNACK- Low-fat milkshake made with: 1 c skim milk, ¾ c fat-free ice cream.

DAY3

BREAKFAST- 2 pancakes, 4in round, 1 tsp fruit spread, or maple spread.

MORNING SNACK- 1 c skim milk, 1 sliced peach.

LUNCH- 1 mixed green salad, 1 tsp fat-free dressing, 6 saltine crackers, 3 oz tuna fish (albacore, water packed), 1 Apple.

AFTERNOON SNACK- ½ oz chocolate (about 4 chocolate kisses).

DINNER- 2 c cooked pasta, ½ c spaghetti sauce with 1 ½ oz cooked ground beef, (lean), 1 mixed green salad, 1 tsp fat-free dressing.

EVENING SNACK- 1 c skim milk, 1 whole graham cracker.

DAY4

BREAKFAST- 1 c orange juice, 1 c cereal, 1 c skim milk, 1 c strawberries.

MORNING SNACK- 2 tsp reduced fat peanut butter, 2 rice cakes.

LUNCH- 1 c veg. soup, 1 mixed green salad, 2 tsp fat-free salad dressing, 1 c skim milk, 6 saltine crackers, 1 oz low-fat mozzarella cheese.

AFTERNOON SNACK- 1 Apple

DINNER-1-piece 5 oz flounder, or other white fish, baked, broiled, or grilled, 1 med. potato, 1 mixed green salad, 1 tsp free salad dressing, 1 c cooked broccoli, 1 whole grain dinner roll.

EVENING SNACK- 3 c lite popcorn.

DAY5

BREAKFAST- 1 English muffin, 1 egg poached, ½ grapefruit,

MORNING SNACK- 1 peach, or other fruit,1 c skim milk, 1c cereal.

LUNCH- 2 oz turkey breast or lean ham, 1 large whole grain pita, 2 boiled sliced carrots, 1 c skim milk.

AFTERNOON SNACK- 1 Pear.

DINNER- 2 slices cheese pizza, 1 big mixed green salad, 1 tsp fat-free salad dressing.

EVENING SNACK- 1 c sliced fruit.

DAY6

BREAKFAST-1 Bagel, 1 tsp lite cream cheese, 1 c orange.

MORNING SNACK- 6 oz, fat-free flavored yogurt.

LUNCH-2 oz lean hamburger, grilled or broiled, 1 tsp ketchup, 1 hamburger bun, ½ tomato sliced, ½ green pepper sliced, 1 c skim milk

DINNER- 2 c angel hair pasta, 3 oz boiled shrimp, 1 tsp olive oil w/garlic on pasta, 1 mixed green salad w/1 tsp fat-free dressing, ½ c cooked green beans, 1 slice Italian bread.

DAY7

BREAKFAST- 1 slice French toast, 1 c fresh blueberries, 1 c skim milk.

MORNING SNACK- 1 Orange.

LUNCH- ½ c cottage cheese, 1 mixed green salad, 1 fat-free dressing, 1 whole wheat roll, 1 c skim milk, 1 c sliced carrots,

AFTERNOON SNACK- 1 oz pretzels,

DINNER- 3 oz baked or broiled cod, 1 ½ c noodles, 2 tsp butter or margarine, 1 c applesauce, 1 c mixed veg.

EVENING SNACK- ½ c fat-free dressing.

2000 Calorie Menu

DAY1

BREAKFAST- 3 plain waffles, 2 tsp maple syrup, 1 tsp butter or margarine, 8 oz water or caffeine-free, non-caloric beverage, ¾ c orange juice.

MORNING SNACK- 1 c skim milk, 1 cinnamon bagel,

LUNCH- Salad w/romaine lettuce, ½ c ea. carrots, green peppers, cabbage, and celery, tsp lite salad dressing, 3 oz turkey breast, 1 whole grain roll.

AFTERNOON SNACK- 1 c sliced strawberries, 6 oz fat-free flavored yogurt, 1 tsp crunchy whole grain cereal,

DINNER- 4 oz sirloin steak, lean only, broiled or grilled without added fat, 1 c rice, 1 tsp butter or margarine, 1 c cooked carrots, 11 mixed green salad, 2 tsp fat-free dressing,

EVENING SNACK- 1 orange.

DAY2

BREAKFAST- 1 c oatmeal, cooked. 1 tsp brown sugar, ¾ c skim milk, 1 c orange juice, 1 slice toast, wheat or rye. 1 tsp butter or margarine.

MORNING SNACK- 1 Apple.

LUNCH- 2 ½ oz turkey breast, mustard, or fat-free mayonnaise, 2 slices whole wheat bread, 1 ½ c sliced cucumbers and carrots, or other raw veg.

AFTERNOON SNACK- ½ c skim milk, 1 c strawberries, 6 vanilla wafer cookies.

DINNER- 4 oz chicken breast, no skin, baked, broiled, or grilled. 1 med. baked potato, 1 tsp butter or margarine, 1 c green beans, 1 mixed green salad, 4 tsp regular Italian salad dressing, 1 whole wheat dinner roll.

EVENING SNACK- Low-fat milkshake made with 1 c skim milk and 1 c fat-free ice cream.

DAY3

BREAKFAST- 3 pancakes, 4" round, 1 tsp fruit spread or maple syrup, 1 c orange juice.

MORNING SNACK- 1 c skim milk, 1 sliced peach.

LUNCH- 1 mixed green salad, 1 tsp fat-free dressing, 1 whole grain dinner roll, 3 oz tuna fish, albacore, water packed, 1 apple.

AFTERNOON SNACK- 1 oz chocolate (about 8 chocolate kisses)

DINNER- 2 ½ c cooked pasta, ½ c spaghetti sauce w/3 oz cooked ground beef, lean, 1 mixed green salad, 1 tsp fat-free dressing.

EVENING SNACK- 1 c skim milk, 1 whole graham cracker.

DAY4

BREAKFAST- 1 c orange juice, 1 ½ c cereal, 1 c skim milk, 1 c strawberries, 2 slices rye or wheat bread, toasted, 2 tsp jelly or jam.

LUNCH- 1 ½ c vegetable soup, 1 mixed green salad, 2 tsp fat-free salad dressing, 1 c skim milk, 1 dinner roll, 1 oz low-fat mozzarella cheese, 6 saltine crackers.

AFTERNOON SNACK- 1 apple.

DINNER-6 oz flounder, or other white fish, baked, broiled, or grilled. 1 med baked potato, 1 mixed green salad, 1 tsp fat-free salad dressing, 1 c cooked broccoli, 1 whole grain dinner roll.

EVENING SNACK- 3 c light popcorn.

DAY5

BREAKFAST- 1 English muffin, 2 tsp jelly or jam, ½ c cholesterol-free egg substitutes, scrambled or 2 egg whites, cooked, ½ grapefruit.

MORNING SNACK- 1 peach or other fruit, 1 c skim milk, 1 ½ c cereal.

LUNCH- 3 oz turkey breast or lean ham, 1 large whole grain pita, 2 sliced carrots, 1 c skim milk.

AFTERNOON SNACK- 1 pear.

DINNER- 3 slices cheese pizza, 1 large mixed green salad, 1 tsp fat-free salad dressing, 1 c mixed fruit.

EVENING SNACK- 3 c light popcorn.

DAY6

BREAKFAST- 1 bagel, 1 tsp light cream cheese, 1 c orange juice.

MORNING SNACK- 6 oz fat-free flavored yogurt, ½ c fresh strawberries.

LUNCH- 3 oz lean hamburger, grilled or broiled, 1 tsp ketchup, 1 hamburger bun, ½ tomato sliced, ½ green pepper, sliced.

AFTERNOON SNACK- 6 vanilla wafers, 1 c skim milk.

DINNER- 3 c angel hair pasta, 4 oz boiled shrimp, 2 tsp olive oil w/garlic on pasta, 1 mixed green salad, 1 tsp fat-free dressing, ½ c cooked green beans, 1 slice Italian bread.

EVENING SNACK- 3 c light popcorn,

DAY7

BREAKFAST-2 slices French toast, 2 tsp butter or margarine, 1 c fresh blueberries, 1 c skim milk.

MORNING SNACK- *1 orange.*

LUNCH- ½ c cottage cheese, 1 mixed green salad, 1 tsp fat-free dressing, 1 whole wheat roll, 1 c skim milk, 1 c sliced carrots.

AFTERNOON SNACK- 1 ¼ oz pretzels.

DINNER- 6 oz baked or broiled cod, 1 ½ c noodles, 1 tsp butter or noodles, 1 c applesauce, 1 c mixed vegetables, 1 mixed green salad, 2 tsp oil, and vinegar dressing.

EVENING SNACK- 1/2 c fat-free pudding.

Chapter Seven: Follow Your Gut

(guthealthproject.com)

Ways to heal your **GUT** naturally (digestive system).

1. *REMOVE FOODS-* Eliminate processed foods with sugar, flour, and vegetable oils.
2. *REPAIR GUT WALL-* Drink bone broth, eat healthy fats like coconut oil, and take cod liver oil supplements.
3. *REBUILD MICROBIOME-* Eat fermented foods like yogurt, kefir, sauerkraut, kombucha, and kimchi every day.
4. *REDUCE STRESS-* Practice meditation, move your body every day and keep a gratitude journal.
5. <u>BONE BROTH</u>- Bone broth is a nutritious broth made from animal's bones (typically chicken, turkey, beef, lamb or fish). The bones are slowly simmered in water for 8+ hours. Many people also add spices and organic vegetables to their bone broth.

Note: *Health Benefits of Bone Broth-* Heals a leaky gut, fights colds and flu, reduces inflammation, reduces joint pain, promotes strong bones, calms and promotes sleep.

Bone Broth (Recipe)
(from MindBodyGreen)

Ingredients

- 1 Organic whole chicken
- 8c water
- 4-6 stalks of celery, finely chopped
- 1/3 white or yellow onion, finely chopped
- 3 cloves garlic, finely chopped
- 1tbsp chopped fresh parsley
- 1-inch ginger root, finely chopped
- ½tsp sea salt
- ½tsp apple cider vinegar

Directions:

Put ingredients in slow cooker and cook on low heat for 8-10 hrs.

Note: You can purchase already prepared Bone Broth in many major stores.

An Unhealthy Gut

(www.carlyonpurpose.com)

Did you know that an 'unhealthy gut' can cause many unpleasant things to happen in your body? For example:

*Constipation/Diarrhea *Bloating/Gas *Food sensitivity *Bad taste in mouth *Foggy or erratic brain *Mood swings *Depression/Fatigue *Headaches, *Skin problems *Auto Immune Disease.

If your **GUT** is sick then you or sick!

The Saliva Test

(www.candidasupport.org)

Your saliva can tell you something about your health. To see if you should cut fungus-promoting foods like cheeses, mushrooms, vinegar, and more. Add more raw garlic to your diet in order to *Heal Your Gut.*

Below is a simple at home "saliva test."

First thing in the morning, place water into a glass and spit into it within 30 min. of waking up. Make sure you do it first thing before you rinse, spit, eat, or drink anything. It takes fifteen minutes for a result. A typical result will show that your saliva will float on the surface, but if the glass is cloudy and your saliva sinks to the bottom of the glass like sediment, you may be seeing colonies of yeast.

Also, if the saliva on top has tiny strings that start to hang down that may look like jellyfish, or you see specks of yeast floating in the middle of the glass, this could also show you have too much yeast in your system.

This is a quick test that you can do at home, but if you are worried, it is always best to visit your local integrative medical practitioner who will be able to take swabs, samples, blood test, and stool tests to check for yeast overgrowth.

Probiotic Supplements

(smarter-reviews.com)

Check out this list of top 5 probiotic supplements of 2018 for 'Gut Health':

1. *Complete Probiotics Platinum (By: 1MD)*
    a. Review ranking 9.6 graded A+/
2. *Pro45 (by: LiveWell)*
    a. Review ranking 8.9, graded B+/
3. *ULTIMATE FLORA, critical care 50 Billion (By: Renew Life)*
    a. Review ranking- 8.6, graded B+/
4. *Culturelle Digestive HealthProbiotic capsules (By: Culturelle)*
    a. Review ranking-7.3, graded C /
5. *TruBiotics Daily Probiotic Supplement (By: (TruBiotics)*
    a. Review ranking- 7.1, graded C-/

Research the above items, and as always:

- **Consult with your doctor** before beginning any over the counter supplements!
- Always purchase at a USDA approved supplements supply store.

What to look for in a good probiotic:

- **"Formulated by a Doctor"** Look for real doctors specializing in gut health backing the product.
- High CFU (**C**olony **F**orming Units) Count: Microbiome is composed of about 100-trillion good and bad bacteria. You should look for a formula with a minimum of 40 billion CFU's
- Multiple "Strains," It is crucial to find probiotics that use a comprehensive approach to promoting balance in your gut bacteria. _Try to find a supplement with **at least 9** individual strains._
- Doesn't Require Refrigeration: You will not always have access to a refrigerator, so choose a probiotic that is well formulated to withstand room temperature and does not require being refrigerated during periods of non-use.

Chicken Clichés to Make You Smile

"What came first, the chicken or the egg?
'Chicken one day, feathers the next,'
'Shush! I'm hatching a plan...'"

Nest egg: Saved money

Hen Party: A gathering of gossiping women

Chicken feed: Small amount of money

What did the hen say when she saw the
scrambled eggs?

O'Cluck', My children are all mixed up!

Flew the coop: Gone

No spring chicken: Getting old

Chapter Eight: Healthier Recipes

Chicken/Dressing (no cornbread)
(Recipe Created by Diane Brown)

Ingredients

- Skinless chicken parts 4-6 pieces
- 1 lg bag frozen broccoli florets
- 1 lg jar Alfredo sauce or 2 cans cream of chicken (your choice)
- 1 bag shredded cheddar cheese

Directions

Bake, boil, or grill chicken. Heat Alfredo sauce on low and cut up chicken pieces into the heated sauce. Steam the frozen ice from the broccoli (completely). Begin to layer the nonstick 9'9 baking pan, broccoli first, then layer with the broccoli and chicken sauce. Top with the complete bag of shredded cheese. Bake at 360 degrees.

This awesome dish replaces my traditional "cornbread dressing!" It's amazing with cranberry sauce! And yes, you can be even more creative and add your choice of additional veggies like onions, red peppers, green peppers, celery, etc. Remember the more you add, the more you should also increase the alfredo sauce.

Enjoy!

Parmesan Chicken Breast

Ingredients

- 8-10 chicken breast
- 2 sticks of margarine, melted (healthy substitute)/ 60-70% vegetable oil spread (butter flavored)
- 1 cup grated parmesan cheese, mixed with seasoned bread crumbs (substitute breadcrumbs with c rolled oats or 1 cup crushed bran cereal).

Directions

Brush chicken with the veg oil spread and roll the chicken in the parmesan mix. Place in baking dish. Bake at 250 degrees for 3 hrs.

Fried Chicken (YES!)

Ingredients

- 2 chicken breasts (less fat), washed
- dry seasonings to your taste.
- ½ pack of *Ritz* crackers (Grind very finely).

Directions

Heat 2-3tbsp canola oil in a skillet, coat chicken breast, and place into heated oil. Fry at med heat. After both sides or browned turn heat even lower, slow cook until done.

Mexican Chicken

Ingredients

- 6 skinless chicken breasts
- Sea salt
- Red pepper
- Garlic powder
- Large bag of Doritos

Ingredients (Sauce)

- 1c Rotel tomatoes
- 1c cream chicken soup
- 1c chicken broth
- 1c chopped green chilies
- ½ onion, chopped

Directions

Mix sauce ingredients together. Set aside.

Preheat oven to 350 degrees and cook 6 skinless chicken breasts (bake, broil, or grill). Cut in pieces, sprinkle with sea salt. Add red pepper and garlic powder.

Mix chicken pieces in with prepared sauce.

In a 9x12 nonstick baking dish, begin layering:

Begin by crushing a couple handfuls of Doritos on the bottom, pour ½ of chicken mixture sauce over the bottom layer of chips, top with broken (not finely crushed) chips again, pour last half of chicken mixture sauce over broken chips.

Top with 1 large bag of shredded cheese, sprinkle a handful of crushed Doritos over the top and bake for 1 hr.

This dish is actually not a bad food choice (If you stick with suggested serving size)! The mixture itself is primarily protein and veggies!

Salads

Salads are a great alternative meal. Keeping salad 'fixings' as a staple in your home is an excellent idea for those times when you are out of time and want something healthy to eat!

Fruitee Salad

Ingredients

- 3 apples, diced
- 3 oranges, diced
- 3 bananas, diced
- 1 small package of sugar-free vanilla pudding
- 1 tub of cool whip
- 1 sm can crushed pineapples (no sugar added), *set juice to the side for later use*
- 1 small jar maraschino cherries (very high in sugar, you may substitute with strawberries)
- ½c reduced sugar orange juice

Directions

Mix the pineapple juice with the orange juice, add the prepared pudding, and ½ or more of cool whip, mix well and stir into diced fruit and crushed pineapples.

Veggie Wraps
(Recipe Created by Diane Brown)

Ingredients

- 1 bundle of leafy green lettuce
- 1 bell pepper (cut in long strips)
- 1 red pepper (cut in long strips)
- 1 pkg green onions (use the darker top portion)
- 1 container veggie ranch dip
- 1 pkg turkey or lean ham strips

Lettuce Prep: Cut lower butt end off, discard, separate leaves, wash, shake excess water off, and dry with paper towel if need.

Directions

Lay an individual leaf out, spread 1-2tbsp ranch dressing in center of the leaf, next lay ½ rolled meat onto spread, next add a strip of red pepper and green onion all centered in the middle of leaf; now, fold each side of leaf lapped over. Tear a piece of plastic cling wrap, carefully lay folded salad wrap onto plastic wrap, wrap plastic around the salad, and leave top exposed for eating. Allow to chill for a couple hrs. or overnight.

Note: 1 lettuce head makes 8-12 Veggie wraps.

Loaded Vegetable Salad
(Recipe Created by Diane Brown)

Ingredients

- 1 head romaine lettuce
- 1 head leafy green lettuce
- purple cabbage
- green onions, broccoli
- bell pepper
- red pepper
- tomatoes
- fresh jalapeños
- shredded cheese
- Imitation bacon bits (30 cal. Per 1 ½ Tbsp)
- boiled eggs
- lean ham/turkey
- 1 crispy bread-n-butter pickle

Directions

How to dress a single salad:

Wash, dry (w/paper towel), and cut up both lettuce heads. Layer a large salad bowl w/purple cabbage, lettuce, meat choice, cheese, another dash of lettuce, peppers, few tomatoes, meat choice, more lettuce, green onions, broccoli, top w/lettuce, tomatoes, sprinkle cheese, boiled egg, top off w/bacon bits, and a crispy bread-n-butter pickle on the side.

Keep-it-simple Caesar Salad

Ingredients

- ¾ head romaine lettuce
- ¼c bacon bits
- ¼c grated parmesan cheese
- 3 tbsp (78 cal. per tbsp) Caesar salad dressing
- Black pepper to taste

Directions

Wash the lettuce and pat dry. Cut or tear the leaves. Mix together the bacon bits, parmesan cheese, and lettuce.

Refrigerate just before serving toss with *fat-free Caesar salad dressing and sprinkle with black pepper.

Apple and Walnut Salad

Ingredients

- 1 celery stalk
- 1c chopped apple
- 1/3c walnut pieces (best nuts for heart health!)
- 2 tbsp vanilla yogurt (choose low-fat or fat-free)

Directions

Wash the celery and cut into 1-inch pieces. In a small bowl, combine the celery with the chopped apple and walnut pieces. Toss with the low-fat yogurt. Serve immediately or cover and chill.

Coleslaw

Ingredients (Slaw)

- 1 bag coleslaw mix
- 1 bell pepper
- 1 container small cherry tomatoes
- 2 cups broccoli

Ingredients (Dressing)

- ½ c low-fat mayonnaise
- 2tbsp white sugar (substitute, 2-3 pkg sweetener)
- 1 ½tbsp lemon juice
- 1tbsp vinegar
- ½tsp black pepper
- ½tsp salt

Directions

Cut up all veggies; you may halve the tomatoes or pour in whole. Toss together the coleslaw mix with the cut up veggies and refrigerate while you prepare the dressing.

Now, whisk mayonnaise, sugar, lemon juice, vinegar, pepper, and salt together in a bowl, until smooth and creamy.

Pour into the veggie mix, toss, serve immediately, or refrigerate for later.

FOOD FOR THOUGHT!

*Cabbage, a Nutritional Powerhouse!

"Cabbage," particularly raw cabbage is one of the healthiest vegetables. Besides being rich in vitamin C, cabbage contains vitamin A, vitamin E, calcium, and folic acid. To gain the greatest nutritional value from cabbage, enjoy it raw! "Losers" have no fear; 1 c of shredded cabbage contains less than 25 calories.

Already Portioned Meatloaves!

Ingredients

- 1 ½ lbs. lean ground beef/chuck
- 1c oats (instead of bread crumbs)
- 1 egg beaten
- 1tsp sea salt
- 1c milk
- ½c chopped green bell pepper

Directions

Mix all together, form into 6-8 small loaves, and place onto a nonstick baking pan. Prepare meatloaf mixture with 1 can cream mushroom soup, 2tsp paprika, and 1 can tomato soup; stir well, and spoon over meatloaf loaves.

Cauliflower and Ground Beef Hash

Ingredients

- 16 oz bag frozen cauliflower, (defrosted and drained)
- 1lb. lean ground beef
- 2 c shredded cheddar cheese
- 1 tsp garlic powder
- salt, and pepper to taste

Directions

Prep: Brown the ground beef over medium heat and drain the grease. Add it back to the pan along with the cauliflower, garlic, salt, and pepper. Cook and stir until the cauliflower is tender. Add cheese on top of the cauliflower and beef mixture. Turn heat to low, cover pan with a lid, and allow cheese to melt.

Cheesy Skillet Taco/ Low Carb

Ingredients

- 1 lb. lean ground beef
- 1 lg yellow onion diced
- 2 bell peppers diced
- 1-12oz can diced tomatoes with green chilies
- 1-2 lg zucchinis, diced
- 2tbsp taco seasoning
- 3c baby kale/spinach mixture
- 1 ½c shredded cheddar and jack cheese
- Green onions to garnish

Directions:

In a large pan, lightly brown ground beef and crumble well. Drain excess fat. Add vegetables and cook until browned. Add canned tomatoes, taco seasoning, and any water needed for taco seasoning to evenly coat mixture. Add greens and let fully wilt. Mix well. Cover with shredded cheese and let cheese melt. When cheese is melted, serve over a bed of lettuce. Garnish with the green onions. 6 servings.

Beef-n-Cabbage Skillet Recipe/ Low Carb

Ingredients

- 1 lb. lean ground beef
- ½ head green cabbage
- 2tbsp unsalted butter
- 3tbsp taco seasoning mix
- ½ diced yellow onion
- 1 ½c shredded 3-cheese blend
- salt, and pepper to taste

Directions

Preheat oven to 350 degrees. In a large skillet, add 1tbsp butter, add shredded cabbage and diced onions, and sauté on medium high heat until the cabbage softens. Remove from the heat and put into a separate dish. In the same skillet, add the remaining tbsps. of butter and cooked ground beef, breaking up meat as it cooks. Add taco seasoning and stir until meat is cooked. Return cabbage to skillet and season with salt and pepper. Fold in a half cup cheese. Top skillet with remaining cheese and place into the oven. Cook until cheese lightly browns.

Crust-less Cheeseburger Quiche

Ingredients

- 1 lb. lean ground beef
- 1-2tsp onion powder
- ½c heavy cream
- ½c mayonnaise
- 3 eggs beaten
- 1c shredded cheddar cheese
- garlic powder to taste, pepper

Directions

Brown ground beef and onion powder in a large skillet over medium heat and drain fat. Mix together eggs, cream, mayonnaise, garlic powder, pepper, and shredded cheese. Put browned beef into a 9in. pie plate; pour remaining ingredients over the beef. Place in a preheated 350-degree oven and bake for 40-45 min. Allow dish to cool slightly, cut and place over chilled lettuce leaves.

Note: Round or Loin are the keywords when looking for the leanest cut of ground beef.

Also, when selecting ground beef, look at the percentages: Ex, 80/20 lean means the meat is 80% lean and 20% fat, preferably look for ground beef labeled 90/10% (or leaner).

*"Where's the Beef"? was introduced in
1984 as a slogan for the fast food chain,
Wendy's

Microwave Vegetarian Lasagna

Ingredients

- ½c crushed tomatoes
- 1/3c ricotta cheese
- 1/3c grated mozzarella cheese
- 1tbsp grated parmesan cheese
- 1/8tsp dried oregano
- 1/8tsp dried basil
- 6 "oven-ready" or pre-cooked lasagna noodles

Directions

Place the crushed tomatoes in a bowl. Stir in the ricotta, then the mozzarella and parmesan. Make sure each cheese is thoroughly mixed in before adding the next. Stir in the oregano and the basil. Lay out 2 lasagna noodles in a large bowl or small ½qt microwave safe casserole dish. Break the noodles to fit into the dish. Spoon approx. 1/3 of the tomato sauce and cheese mixture evenly over the top. Repeat the layering 2 more times. Cover the dish with wax paper; microwave on high heat for 3 min. Turn the bowl, microwave on high heat for another 3-5 min. until the cheese is cooked. Let stand for 10 min. before serving.

Vegetarian Cabbage Rolls

Ingredients

- 6oz firm tofu
- 2tsp olive oil
- 1 garlic clove
- ½ red onion
- 1c crushed tomatoes
- ½ green bell pepper
- ½ tsp ground cumin
- 1/8tsp (or to taste) paprika
- 8-10 boiled cabbage leaves
- 6oz tomato sauce
- 3oz water
- 2tbsp white vinegar
- 2tsp granulated sugar

Directions

Preheat oven to 350 degrees. Spray a large baking sheet with nonstick cooking spray. Drain the tofu and dice into small pieces. Heat the olive oil in a medium sized frying pan. Add the garlic and red onion. Sauté until the onion is tender. Crumble the tofu into the frying pan. Add the tomatoes and green pepper, mashing the tomatoes with a spatula to break them up slightly. Stir in the ground cumin and paprika.

Lay a cabbage leaf flat on the counter. Spread 2 heaping tbsps of filling in the middle. Roll up the bottom, tuck in the sides, and continue rolling up to the top. Place the roll in the baking dish with the steamed section on the bottom. In a small bowl, mix together the tomato sauce, water, white vinegar, and sugar. Pour over the cabbage rolls.

Place the dish in the oven and bake the cabbage rolls for 40-45 minutes.

Hearty Vegetarian Egg Drop Soup

Ingredients

- 1 garlic clove
- 1 zucchini
- 2 Roma tomatoes
- 1tsp olive oil
- 4c low sodium vegetable broth
- ¼tsp salt
- 1/8tsp black pepper
- ½tsp dried basil
- 2tbsp egg substitute

Directions

Smash, peel, and chop the garlic clove. Wash the zucchini, peel, and cut into thin slices. Wash and dice the tomatoes. Heat the olive oil in a med. size saucepan over medium-low to medium heat. Add the garlic and the diced tomato, stirring. Cook for a few minutes; then, add the zucchini. Add the broth and bring to a boil. Stir in the salt, pepper, and dried basil. Cook for another 2-3min. Turn off the heat, stir in the egg substitute, and serve.

Broccoli Baked Potato

Ingredients

- 4 russet potatoes
- Olive oil

Ingredients (sauce)

- ½ lb. frozen broccoli florets
- 3tbsp butter
- 3tbsp all-purpose flour
- 3c whole milk
- ½tsp salt
- ¼tsp garlic powder
- 6oz medium shredded cheddar cheese

Directions

Prepare 4 russet potatoes, wash, and coat each with olive oil; place the oil covered potato on a baking sheet, and season generously with salt. Bake the potatoes in a preheated oven at 400 degrees for 45-60 min. or until tender all the way through. As the potatoes are baking, prepare the sauce.

Directions (Broccoli Cheese Sauce)

Allow the broccoli to thaw, chop into small pieces, and set aside until ready to use. Add the butter and flour to a medium saucepan; place the pan over a medium flame. Whisk the butter and flour together as they melt.

Allow the mixture to begin to bubble and foam, whisking continuously. Continue to cook for 1 min. to remove the raw flour flavor, but do not let the flour begin to brown. Whisk the milk into the butter and flour mixture. Bring the milk up to a simmer, whisking frequently. When it reaches a simmer, it will thicken.

Once thick enough to coat a spoon, turn the heat down to the lowest setting. Season the white sauce with the salt and garlic powder. Add a handful of the shredded cheese to the sauce at a time, whisking until it has fully melted before you add the next handful. Once all the cheese has been melted into the sauce, stir in the chopped broccoli.

Keep on low heat and stir occasionally. After the potatoes are finished baking, take them out and carefully cut partially down the middle, while slightly mashing the insides of each potato. Afterward, dip ladles of broccoli cheese sauce over each potato. Garnish with extra shredded cheddar, if desired.

Banana Pancakes (Gluten-Free, Flourless, Low-Calorie)

Ingredients

- 1 ½ large bananas, ripe-overripe
- 2 eggs
- 1/8 tsp baking powder
- maple syrup
- butter, or blueberries to serve

Directions

In a large mixing bowl, crack in the eggs. Add baking powder; whisk to combine. In another bowl, add the bananas. Lightly mash w/fork (not too much). Pour the egg mixture into the partially mashed bananas; stir to combine. In a sprayed frying pan, cook mini pancakes (1/4 cup).

When the baking powder is activated, flip it over and cook for an additional min.

Serve immediately while hot.

Meatless Burgers

Veggie Burger, Tofu Burger, Portobello Burger, Eggplant Hummus Burger, Beet Burger, Bean and Zucchini Cutlets, Baked Broccoli Burger, Lentil Cauliflower Burger, Best Black Bean Veggie Burger, Martha Stewart's Veggie Burger.

Smoothies
(Listotic.com)

Smoothies have become not only healthy but an excellent meal replacement during a time when most of us live in the 'fast lane,' and there's no time for traditional meals. If made with health in mind, you've got your vitamins, minerals, fiber, and protein in this one drink!

1. Morning Magic-1c cold coffee, 1 frozen banana, 1/3c plain yogurt, 1 scoop protein powder, 1tbsp flax-meal, ice as desired.
2. Detox- ½ frozen banana, 1c spinach, 2-3tbsp lemon juice, 1tbsp fresh ginger, ¼c blueberries, ¼c cucumbers, 1/2c coconut water
3. Anti-bloat: ½c coconut water, 1 frozen banana, ½ cucumber, 1-2tbsp fresh ginger, 1tsp apple cider vinegar(optional), ice as desired.
4. Kick Starter- ½c blueberries, ½ frozen banana, 1 peeled carrot, 2tbsp Rolled oats, 1tbsp flax-meal, 1c almond milk, ice as desired.

5. Very Berry- 1c frozen berries, ½ frozen banana, 1c spinach, ½c plain yogurt, 1c coconut milk, 1tbsp flax-meal, ice as desired.

6. Chocolate Almond- 1 frozen banana, 1-2tbsp almond butter, 1c almond milk, 1tbsp cacao powder, a dash of sea salt, ice as desired.

7. Cinnamon Roll- ¼c rolled oats, ½c plain yogurt, 1c almond milk, a sm handful pecans, 1 frozen banana, ¼tsp vanilla, ½tsp cinnamon, ice as desired.

8. Apple Pie- ½ lg apple, ½ frozen banana, small handful pecans, 1c almond milk, ¼tsp vanilla, ½tsp cinnamon, ice as desired.

Weight Loss Smoothies
(stylecraze.com)

1. Orange, Lemon, and Flax Seed Smoothie- 2 lg oranges, 2tbsp lemon juice, 1tbsp ground flax seeds, a pinch of Himalayan pink salt Prep: peel the oranges, take out the seeds, and roughly chop them. Toss the chopped oranges into a blender, add lemon juice, and ground the flax seeds. Blend it well and pour out the smoothie into a glass. Add a pinch of Himalayan pink salt and stir well before drinking.

2. Blueberry, Oats, and Chia Smoothie- ½c blueberries, ¼c oats, 2tbsp chia seeds, 2c low-fat milk. Prep: Blend the blueberries, oats, chia seeds, and the milk. Pour the smoothie out into two glasses and enjoy!

3. Cucumber, Plum, and Cumin Smoothie- 2c cucumber, ½c plum, 1tsp cumin powder, 1tbsp lime juice, a pinch of Himalayan pink salt. Prep: Toss the cucumber and plum into a blender and give it a spin. Pour the smoothie out into two glasses and add cumin powder, lime juice, and a pinch of Himalayan pink salt. Stir well before drinking.

Smoothie Tips

1. A "QUALITY BLENDER" is a must-have!

2. Use frozen fruit instead of ice. This makes for a thicker consistency. *Easy cleaning blender method, rinse it, refill it half full of hot water and a little detergent, turn the blender on, and allow it to clean itself.

3. Cucumbers are low in calories and high in water content.

4. Plums help fight cancer.

5. Cumin seeds can help improve digestion.

6. Limes contain d-limonene, a terpene that helps prevent cancer.

7. Blueberries are rich in fiber.

8. Oats are a great source of dietary fiber that aids weight loss.

9. Green Apples contain antioxidants such as catechin, quercetin, chlorogenic acid, etc. that aid weight loss, prevent asthma attacks, and prevent cancer and cardiovascular disease.

10. Ginger helps improve digestion and delays aging

Tips For The Holidays!

*Don't skip Breakfast

*Turkey or Chicken Broth: Fresh boiled poultry should be placed in the refrigerator overnight so that excess fat can be skimmed off of broth.

*Season broth with chicken bouillon or any other choice poultry seasoning. This is an excellent way to eliminate saturated fats while adding essentially no fat!

*A couple of hours before dinner, eat a small salad and drink a refreshing glass of lemon water. This prevents over indulging at dinner!

*At dinner, load up on veggies, have a moderate amount of white meat(s), and limit yourself to one serving of other entrees.

*Dessert: Pick out a couple of your favorites and eat a half serving of each.

Note: Ice-box desserts are less fattening than cakes and oven baked pies. Beware of the sugar content in some of these type desserts.

*Eat slow. Conversate. Enjoy the family!

*Leftovers: Don't have any! Prepare just enough for the day's dinner.

Have A Healthy Holiday

Chapter Nine: Food for Thought

("giving thanks" Publishers Inc. and www.everything.com)

*Never put potatoes in the refrigerator. Why? The cold temperature will turn its starch into sugar more quickly, instead put them into a paper bag and store in a cool place not cold.

*A slice of soft bread placed in the package of hardened, brown sugar or hard cookies, will soften them in a couple of hours.

*No more tears when peeling onions if you place them in the deep freeze for 4 or 5 min. first.

*Vinegar brought to a boil in a new frying pan, will prevent foods from sticking.

*Muffins will slide right out of tin pans if the hot pan is first placed on a wet towel.

*A few drops of lemon juice added to simmering rice will keep the grains separate.

*If you've over-salted soup or vegetables, add cut raw potatoes, and discard once they have cooked and absorbed the salt.

*If you've over-sweetened a dish, add salt.

*Drop a lettuce leaf into a pot of homemade soup to absorb excess grease from the top.

*If fresh vegetables are wilted or blemished, pick off the brown edges, sprinkle with cold water, wrap in paper towel, and refrigerate for an hour or so.

*Lettuce and celery keep longer if you store them in paper bags, instead of cellophane.

*Brown sugar will not harden if an apple slice is placed in the container

*Thaw fish in milk. The milk draws out the frozen taste and provides a fresh-caught flavor.

*Chop- to cut food into small pieces.

*Dice- to cut food into small cubes no larger than ¼ inch.

*Drain- to remove water from blanched, washed rinse, or boiled food.

*Marinate- to soak food in a liquid before cooking both to tenderize it and add flavor. Most marinades contain an acidic ingredient such as lemon juice, wine, or vinegar.

*Blanch- To purge vegetables and other food briefly into boiling water. Blanching seals in colors and textures of tender-crisp vegetables. Blanched foods that aren't going to be cooked immediately should be dipped into ice-cold water. This "shocks" the food and stops the cooking process.

*The freshness of eggs can be tested by placing them in a large bowl of cold water. If they float, "**DO NOT USE THEM."**

*For a juicier hamburger, add cold water to the beef, before grilling (½c to 1 lb. meat).

*To keep cauliflower white while cooking, add a little milk to the water.

7 Days of Challenges

Sometimes it's the 'challenge' of a task that can motivate or 'jump start' our desire to make a healthy change in our lives.

Use this challenge to get YOU started!

Monday	Go 'meatless'
Tuesday	Walk-A-Mile
Wednesday	Water-up (drink at least 8, 8 oz glasses)
Thursday	Sugarless (eliminate sugar!)
Friday	Read-A-Book
Saturday	Take a 'tub' bath
Sunday	Attend Sunday School (or bible study)

What is the life expectancy of your workout shoes?

Most running shoes will last up to 500 miles. If you know on average what you typically run/walk, simply add your weekly workout miles. If you have an active average workout routine, you can typically expect a 6-month lifespan.

Tip: If you wear your shoes for exercise time only (not as daily wear), they will last longer.

Did You Also Know?

5K= 3.1 miles

10K= 6.22 miles

Half Marathon= 13.1 miles

Marathon= 26.2 miles

Recipe for a Happy Marriage
(etsy.com)

Ingredients

- 4c love
- 2c loyalty
- dash of faith
- 3c kindness
- 4c understanding
- 1c friendship
- 5 Spoonfuls of hope
- 1 barrel of laughter
- a pinch of forgiveness (no substitutions)
- Dash of Thoughtfulness (not optional)

Directions

Take love and loyalty and mix thoroughly with faith. Blend in kindness and understanding, add friendship and hope, and sprinkle abundantly with laughter. Garnish with forgiveness and thoughtfulness. Bake with sunshine. Serve daily with generous helpings.

Obituary For Pillsbury Doughboy

Dear Friends,

It is with the saddest heart that I pass on the following. Please join me in remembering a great icon. The Pillsbury Doughboy died yesterday of a yeast infection and complications from repeated pokes in the belly. He was 71. Doughboy was buried in a lightly greased coffin. Dozens of celebrities turned out to pay their respects, including Mrs. Butterworth, Hungry Jack, the California Raisins, Betty Crocker, the Hostess Twinkies, and Cap'n Crunch.

The gravesite was piled high with flours as a long-time friend, Aunt Jemima, delivered the eulogy, describing Doughboy as a man who never knew how much he was kneaded. Doughboy rose quickly in show business, but his later life was filled with turnovers. He was not considered a very smart cookie; wasting much of his dough on half-baked schemes. Despite being a little flaky at times, he (even still as a crusty old man), was considered a roll model for millions.

Toward the end, it was thought he would rise again, but alas, he was no tart. Doughboy is survived by his wife, Play Dough and two children, John Dough and Jane Dough; plus, they had one in the oven.

He is also survived by his elderly father, Pop Tart. The funeral was held at 3:50 for about 20 min.

Tom Anthony's Math:

Did you know there was a formula for computing years of life gained after age 40?

Running for 2hrs a week should gain you about 4 years of life. So that is roughly 100 hours per year for your remaining 40 years or 4000 hours in total for all 40 years.

In one year, there or 24hr/dayx365 days= 8.760 hrs.

So, 4 additional yrs. Is 8,760 hour/year x 4 year= 35,040 hours of life gained.

To gain these extra hours you expended 4,000 hours of running. So, the payback ratio is 35,040 hours gain/ 4,000 hrs. expended= 8.8.

So, running for an hour gives you 9 hours of *extra* life!

The Healthy Plate

Like your meals, your plate should be 'balanced' with a healthy mixture of food groups!

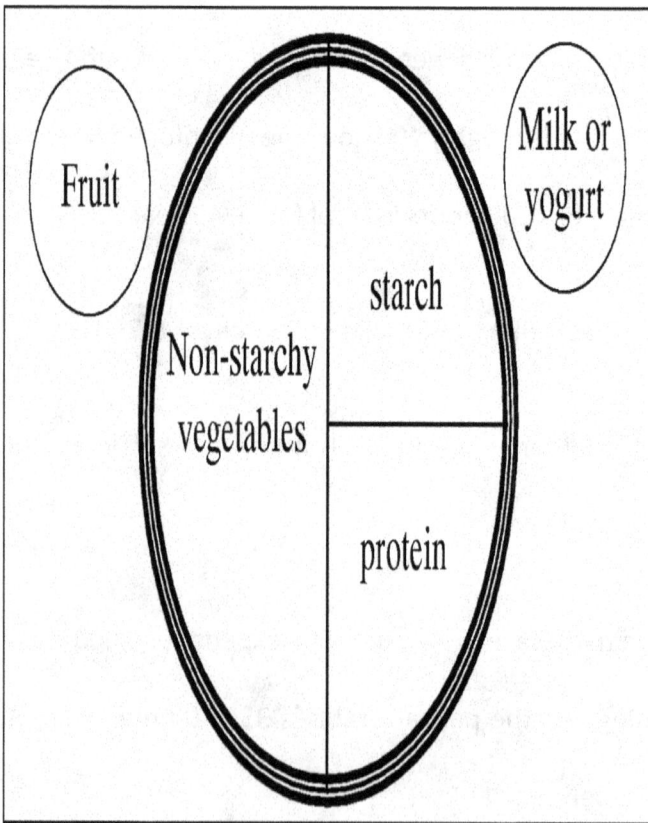

Chapter Ten: Scrambled Facts

(Preventions: Lose Weight 1994 Guidebook)

Sweets
(Gaurdyourhealth.com)

Did you know?

Consuming more than 9 tsp of sugar a day for men and 6 tsp for women can lead to health problems such as tooth decay, obesity, and depression.

There are two types of sugar: *Natural sugar* found in (fruits, milk, and some whole grains) and *Added sugar* (fructose corn syrup) which is added to processed foods and drinks such as cookies, cereal, and soda.

Here are a few ways sugar affects the body:

BRAIN- Added sugar can be as addictive as drugs, tobacco, or alcohol. It affects the same regions of the brain triggering the pleasure sensors to release "dopamine" (makes you want to eat more even when you are not hungry).

LIVER- When you consume too much *added sugar*, your liver has to work extra hard to process it (Attributes to "Diabetes"). *Excess* sugar in the liver often turns into *fat*.

PANCREAS- Too much added sugar in the body can overload and damage your pancreas. The pancreas controls the blood sugar called insulin that powers your muscles and organs. Lack of insulin can cause muscle and nerve damage.

Limit added sugars in your diet by making healthier choices: Reach for fresh fruit instead of pie, donuts, or cake. *Bring your own healthy snacks (frozen grapes, trail mix, yogurt, almonds, peanut butter, and celery sticks, and or apple slices) to work.

Note: Eat a smaller serving of sweet treats, such as a snack-size candy bar, rather than a full-size.

The Benefits Of Chocolate
(When consumed in moderation)

1) Improve blood pressure

2) Improve cholesterol

3) Reduce the risk of cardiovascular disease

4) Enhance brain function

5) Lower stress level

Skinny Chunky Monkey Cookies

Ingredients

- 3 ripe bananas
- 2c old fashioned oats
- 1/4c creamy peanut butter
- 1/4c unsweetened cocoa powder
- 1/2c unsweetened applesauce
- 2-4tbsp of honey
- a dash of cinnamon (optional)
- 1tsp vanilla extract
- 1/4c mini semi-sweet chocolate chips (optional)

Directions

Preheat oven to 350 degrees. Mash bananas in a large bowl and stir in remaining ingredients. Let batter stand for approx. 20 min. then drop by a heaping *"Teaspoon"* onto ungreased cookie sheet. Bake 10-12min.

(These cookies retain their shape and don't spread out on the cookie sheet). Minus the chocolate chips in this recipe, each cookie (1 cookie) equals approximately 56 calories. (sixsistersstuff.com)

75 CALORIE CUPCAKES

Ingredients

- 1 box angel food cake mix
- water
- 1 carton Cool Whip (heavy cream version is super low carb)
- Fresh strawberries (cut into quarters, with no added sugars or gels)
- cupcake liners

Directions

Preheat oven to 350 degrees. Prepare angel food according to instructions. Spoon the batter into the cupcake liners about ¾ full (will make about 41 cupcakes).

Bake for 8 min. until the top is slightly colored. Allow to cool completely. Add 2tbsp Cool Whip to ea. cupcake.

Top with cut up fresh strawberries.

BAKED APPLES

Ingredients

- 1 Apple
- 1tsp brown sugar
- ½ tsp butter
- a pinch of cinnamon

Directions

Wash, slice, and peel the apple. Place apple in a microwave bowl. Sprinkle brown sugar and cinnamon over apples. Top with butter. Microwave on high for 2 minutes. You may top with Cool Whip or sugar-free ice-cream (both optional).

LOW-CALORIE BANANA PUDDING

Ingredients

- 1 box sugar-free vanilla pudding
- 2-3 bananas
- 1 container Cool Whip
- ½ box vanilla wafers

Directions

Prepare vanilla pudding according to box instructions (refrigerate). Slice bananas, crush ½ the bag of vanilla wafers. After pudding has set, fold in ¼ of the container of Cool Whip and fluff them together. Spread the pudding mixture evenly into a med. size (9'5 inch) dessert dish. Layer bananas on top of the vanilla mix. Spread the remaining cool whip over bananas. Complete by sprinkling crushed wafers over top of pudding.

STRAWBERRY BANANA ICE- CREAM

Ingredients

- 1 banana peeled, cut into chunks and frozen
- 3/4c frozen strawberries

Directions

Place the frozen banana and strawberries into a food processor or blender and pulse until smooth. Scrape down the sides as necessary. Serve immediately for a soft-serve consistency or place it in an air-tight container and freeze for a couple of hours to get a *scoop-able* texture.

Enjoy!

(Aseasyasapplepie.com)

Lapses

Lapses are inevitable; most dieters have experienced peaks of joy and valleys of distress. It is the rare person who has not eaten some high-calorie foods, overeaten at a special event or holiday gathering, or resorted to their favorite foods when times get tough. The issue is not so much whether the lapses occur, but the dieter's reaction after they occur.

Below are specific steps that can help:

1. **Stop, Look, and Listen.** A lapse is a signal of impending danger. **Stop** what you are doing, especially if the lapse has started and examine the situation. What is occurring? Why is a lapse in progress? Consider removing yourself to a safe location where you won't be tempted and where you can think rationally.

2. **Stay Calm.** If you get anxious or blame yourself for the lapse, the situation may get worse. A lapse does

not prove a failure. Keeping a cool head makes the following three steps easier.

3. **Renew Your Diet Vows.** Take a minute to remind yourself of how far you have come, the progress you have made, and how sad it would be if one lapse canceled out all your hard work. Restate your program goals and renew the vows you made when dieting began.

4. **Analyze the Lapse.** Instead of blaming yourself for letting go, use the situation to learn what places you at risk. Do certain feelings create the risk? Is it the presence of food, others eating, or other activities? Did you do anything to defend yourself against the urge? Did it work?

5. **Take Charge Immediately.** Leap into action! Leave the house and feed the remaining food to the disposal or do whatever works for you.

More Scrambled Facts

Water-Facts
(www.watercoolersdirect.com)

*2 8oz glasses of water upon waking up: helps activate internal organs. *1 glass of water 30 min. before a meal: aids digestion and cuts back on food consumption. *1 glass of water before taking a bath: helps lower blood pressure. *1 glass of cold water before going to bed is said to lessen the chance of stroke or heart attack: allows your body to relax instead of working harder to replenish you with necessary nutrients

Flat Tummy Water
(stepintomygreenworld.com)

- 6c filtered water
- 1tbsp grated ginger
- 1 cucumber sliced
- 1/3c mint leaves.

Allow the mixture to infuse overnight. Drink it all the next day.

A Few Orange-Facts
(www.healthpositiveinfo.com)

Oranges prevent cancer, lower cholesterol, lower high blood pressure, cardiovascular benefits, treat arthritis, proper brain development, keep sperm healthy, strengthen the immune system, prevent kidney stones, promote weight loss, maintain healthy skin, protects against infections, relieve constipation, maintain bone and teeth health, and prevent ulcers.

Lemon Water Benefits
(Dr. Axe "Food is Medicine)

1. Aids in digestion and detoxification
2. Helps you shed pounds
3. Increases the vitamin C quotient
4. Boosts energy and mood
5. Rejuvenates skin and body healing

Vitamin Sense
(Mayo Clinic Health)

"Supplements are not substitutes." They can't replace the hundreds of nutrients in whole foods that you need for a nutritionally balanced diet.

However, if you do decide to take a vitamin or mineral supplement, here are some factors to consider:

Avoid supplements that provide "megadoses."

In general, choose a multivitamin-mineral supplement that provides about 100% DV of all the vitamins and minerals instead of one that supplies, for example, 500%DV of one vitamin and only 20%DV of another. The exception of this is calcium.

You may notice that calcium-containing supplements don't provide 100%DV. If they did, the tablet would be too large to swallow. (You would simply double the dose, in order to get your 100% Daily Dose). However, having the balance of vitamins and minerals in your body is essential.

Prolonged vitamin or mineral deficiencies can cause specific diseases or conditions such as:

- Night blindness (vitamin A deficiency)
- Pernicious anemia (vitamin B-12 deficiency)
- Anemia (iron deficiency)

Too much of some vitamins and minerals can cause toxic reactions.

The ABC's of Vitamins

Do you know how essential vitamins are and why?

A- Eyes, Immune System, Skin.

B6- Brain Function, Nerve Function, Red cell production.

B12- Red Cell Production, Nerve Function.

C- Bones, Teeth, Skin.

D- Bones, Calcium Absorption.

E- Red Blood Cell Damage,

Folic Acid- Cell Health, Heart Disease.

K- Blood Clotting,

Niacin- Promotes Conversion of food to Energy.

Riboflavin- Energy, Chemical Processes.

Chapter Eleven: Miscellaneous

Standard Cooking Measurements
Measurements Conversion Chart

US Dry Volume Measurements

Measure	Equivalent
1/16 teaspoon	Dash
1/8 teaspoon	A pinch
3 teaspoons	1 tablespoon
1/8 cup	2 tablespoons
1/4 cup	4 tablespoons
1/3 cup	5 tablespoons + 1 tsp
¾ cup	12 tablespoons
1 cup	16 tablespoons
1 pound	16 ounces

US Liquid Volume Measurements

8 Fluid ounces	1 cup
1 pint	2 cups (=16 fluid oz)
1 Quart	2 pints (=4 cups)
1 Gallon	4 quarts (=16 cups)

US to Metric Conversions

1/5 teaspoon	1 ml (milliliter)
1 teaspoon	5 ml
1 fluid oz	30 ml
1/5 cup	50 ml
1 cup	240 ml
2 cups (1 pint)	470 ml
4 cups (1 quart)	.95 liter
4 quarts (1 gal.)	3.8 liter
1 oz	28 grams
1 pound	458 grams

Common Food and Their Calorie Count

myfoodbuddy.com and cookbook publishers, inc.

Almonds, Roasted In Oil, Salted 9-10 Nuts 62 Cal.	Flour (All Purpose) 1c 419 Cal
Angel Food Cake 1 Slice 125 Cal.	Flour (Buckwheat) 1c 326 Cal
Apple Juice 1 Cup 115 Cal	Frankfurters, All Meat (1) 133 Cal
Apple Pie 1 Slice 405 Cal	Graham Cracker (Plain) 2 60 Cal
Apple (Med Size) 95 Cal	Ground Beef, Lean 3oz 230 Cal
Baking Powder Biscuit (1) 95 Cal	Honey 1tbsp 65 Cal
Blueberries (Fresh) 1 Cup 80 Cal	Honey Nut Cheerios, 1oz 105 Cal

Bolonga, 2 Silices 180 V	Ice Cream, Vanilla (11%) 3oz 100 Cal
Brazil Nuts (1oz) 185 Cal	Ice-Cream, Vanilla (Soft Serve,3%) 1c 225 Cal
Broccoli, Frozen, Cooked, 1c, Drained 50 Cal	Jello 1tbsp 50 Cal
Brown-N-Serve Sausage 1 Link 50 Cal	Kale, Cooked from Raw, 1c 40 Cal
Butter, Salted 1tbsp 100 Cal	Lettuce (Loose Leaf) 1c 10 Cal
*Butter, Unsalted 1tbsp *100	Lobster (Cooked in Shell) 1lb 112 Cal
Bacon, Fried (2med Slices) 86 Cal	Lobster, Cooked Or Canned (Meat Only) 69 Cal
Bacon (Canadian) Fried, 1 Slice 58 Cal	Mayonnaise (Imitation) 1 Tbsp 35 Cal

Banana 1 Avg. 118	Mayonnaise (Regular) 1tbsp 100 Cal
Baked Beans ½ c 156	Mixed Grain Bread, 1 Slice 65 Cal
Beans (Green) ½ c 22	Nature Valley Cereal, 1oz 125 Cal
Cooked Cabbage (1 Cup) 30	Orange, 1 60 Cal
Carrot Cake/W Frosting 1 Slice 385 Cal	Pancake (Plain from Mix) 1 60 Cal
Cheddar Cheese, 1oz (Slice) 115 Cal	Peach (Fresh) 1 Avg. 38 Cal
Cheeseburger 4oz Patty 525 Cal	Pecan Pie, 1 Slice 575 Cal
Chicken Breast (Fried) 3.5oz 220 Cal	Pizza (Cheese), 1 Slice 290 Cal

*Chicken Breast (Roasted) 3.0oz *140 Cal	Popcorn, in Veg. Oil (salted) 1c 55 Cal
Chili W/Beans ½C 170 Cal	Quiche Lorraine, 1 Slice 600 Cal
Corn, Drained Whole Kernel ½C 69 Cal	Raisin Bran, 1oz 90 Cal
Cucumber 6 Slices 5 Cal	Raisin Bread, 1 Slice 65 Cal
Danish Pastry Plain (No Nuts) 1oz 110 Cal	Raisins, 1 Pkg 40 Cal
Egg, (Fried) 1 90 Cal	Rice (White) Cooked 1c 225 Cal
*Egg, (Boiled) 1 *82 cal	Salmon (smoked) 3oz 150 cal
Strawberries, fresh whole, ½c 28 cal	Tomatoes, ripe, 1 20 cal

Tuna (in oil), drained ½c 158 cal	Tuna (water packed) 4oz 144 cal
Vegetables, mixed, canned, 1 75 cal	Vienna sausage, 1 45 cal
Walnuts (English) 1oz 180	Wheat bread, 1 slice 65 cal
Wine, (red) 3.5oz 75 cal	Yogurt w/low-fat milk, plain 8oz 145 cal
Yogurt w/nonfat milk, 8oz 125 cal	Yogurt w/whole milk 8oz 140 cal
Zucchini, ½c 16 cal	

ZERO CALORIE FOODS!

Each of these foods has fewer than 52 calories per 100-gram serving:

Cucumber 16 cal.

Celery 16 cal.

Tomatoes 17 cal.

Zucchini 17 cal.

Asparagus 20 cal.

Cauliflower 25 cal.

Cabbage 25 cal.

Turnips 28 cal.

Lemons 29 cal.

Watermelon 30 cal.

Broccoli 34 cal.

Mushrooms 38 cal.

Onions 40 cal.

Carrots 41 cal.

Grapefruit 42 cal.

Beets 43 cal.

Brussels Sprouts 43 cal.

Oranges 47 cal.

Kale 49 cal. Apple 52 cal.

THESE FOODS CAN BE EATEN WITH NO LIMITS! NO PORTION CONTROL! ENJOY!

"EAT THIS, NOT THIS"
(CROSSFITPROPER.COM /Pinterest)

There are some foods that you can easily substitute that will be very beneficial to your health.

Review the next few pages for suggestions on how to make dietary changes that will enhance your weight loss efforts.

Sweet potato fries or mashed sweet potatoes **NOT THIS** French fries/Potatoes	Cauliflower Rice **NOT THIS** White Rice	Zucchini spaghetti **NOT THIS** Pasta/Noodles
Frozen fruit **NOT THIS** Ice Cream	Almond Coconut Milk **NOT THIS** Dairy	Wine (8oz or less), Tequila **NOT THIS** Alcohol
Ghee/Kerrygold Butter **NOT THIS** Butter	White meat turkey breast **NOT THIS** Dark turkey meat	1 Dinner Roll **NOT THIS** Cornbread
Pumpkin Pie **NOT THIS** Pecan Pie	Wheat, whole grain, or multigrain **NOT THIS** White bread	Fat-Free milk, 1% **NOT THIS** whole, or 2%

Vegetable, canola, or olive oils, spray oils **NOT THIS** butter, margarine, lard	Fresh, frozen, or canned fruit in its own juice **NOT THIS** Canned fruit in heavy/ lite syrup	Fresh fruit, Graham or animal crackers **NOT THIS** cookies, cakes, chips
Water, diet soda, seltzer **NOT THIS** soda and other drinks w/sugar	Low salt turkey, grilled chicken, lean **NOT THIS** hot dogs, spam, bologna, salami	1 c steel cut Oats w/0 sugar **NOT THIS** ½ c granola
2 slices whole grain toast **NOT THIS** 1 plain bagel (1 avg. sz bagel = 300 calories)	½c berries (sugar, 5) **NOT THIS** 1c fruit juice (sugar,21)	1 whole grain English muffin (132 calories) **NOT THIS** 1 blueberry muffin (444 calories)

Dried fruit **NOT THIS** Sweet candy	Dark Chocolate (70%) **NOT THIS** Milk Chocolate	Rolled Oats **NOT THIS** Breadcrumbs
Almond Flour **NOT THIS** All-purpose flour	Brown Rice **NOT THIS** White rice	Sea Salt **NOT THIS** Iodine table salt
Oil & Vinegar/salsa **NOT THIS** Salad dressing		

Debt-Loss
(52 Week Money Challenge Sheet)

52 Week Money Challenge

Keep this chart in a place you look at every day so that you can track your savings progress using its simple program. Deposit the recommended amount each week and mark it in the "Deposit Complete" column.

Set up your personalized Savings Account with a Member Advisor today and begin saving with just $1!

Week	Deposit Amount	Deposit Complete	Account Balance	Week	Deposit Amount	Deposit Complete	Account Balance
1	$1		$1	27	$27		$378
2	$2		$3	28	$28		$406
3	$3		$6	29	$29		$435
4	$4		$10	30	$30		$465
5	$5		$15	31	$31		$496
6	$6		$21	32	$32		$528
7	$7		$28	33	$33		$561
8	$8		$36	34	$34		$595
9	$9		$45	35	$35		$630
10	$10		$55	36	$36		$666
11	$11		$66	37	$3*		$703
12	$12		$78	38	$38		$741
13	$13		$91	39	$39		$780
14	$14		$105	40	$40		$820
15	$15		$120	41	$41		$861
16	$16		$136	42	$42		$903
17	$17		$153	43	$43		$946
18	$18		$171	44	$44		$990
19	$19		$190	45	$45		$1,035
20	$20		$210	46	$46		$1,081
21	$21		$231	47	$47		$1,128
22	$22		$253	48	$48		$1,176
23	$23		$276	49	$49		$1,225
24	$24		$300	50	$50		$1,275
25	$25		$325	51	$51		$1,326
26	$26		$351	52	$52		$1,378

*The 52 week Money Challenge was developed by Kassondra Perry-Moreland. Find it also on Facebook at Kassondra's 52 Week Money Challenge.

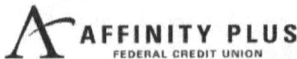

AFFINITY PLUS
FEDERAL CREDIT UNION
Open your savings account online at www.affinityplus.org!

Chapter Twelve: Brain Foods
(Eliminate Stress)

Some say an apple a day can keep the doctor away. I agree. But I also think in addition to diet and exercise that you must maintain your emotional health too. One way to reduce stress is to laugh.

FUN WITH NUMBERS

Think of any number.

Subtract 1 from the number you have thought of.

Multiply that number by 3.

Add 12. Divide that number by 3.

Add 5.

Subtract the original number you thought of from that answer.

(Check your number with the number on page 206)

Think of a number.

Double it.

Add ten.

Half it.

Take away the number you started with.

(Check your number with the number on page 206)

JUST FOR FUN!

What building has the most stories?

What can be swallowed, but can also swallow you?

What can clap without any hands?

A woman has seven children, half of them are boys.
How is this possible?

The 22nd and 24th presidents of the U.S. had the same
parents but were not brothers. How can this be possible?

What has no weight, but is heavy enough to sink a ship?

My friend can shave over ten times a day but still has a full beard. How can this be possible?

The mayor of the city has a brother. His name is John. John says he doesn't have a brother.
How can this be possible?

Work this without a calculator or paper, just your mind:
You have 1000, add 40, add 1000, add 30, again 1000, add 20, add again 1000, and finally 10.
What is the result?
Did you say 5000? You're wrong. It's 4100!
(Now check with a calculator)

Can you find the the mistake 1 2 3 4 5 6 7 8 9 10?

(Answers are on page 206 and 207)

Ten Fun Facts

1) You can't wash your eyes with soap.

2)You can't count your hair.

3)You can't breathe through your nose with your tongue out.

4)You just tried #3!

6) When you did #3 you realized it's possible, only you look like a dog!

7) You're smiling right now because you were fooled.

8) You skipped #5.

9) You just checked to see if there is a #5.

10) Share this with your friends to have some fun too!

Only Great Minds Can Read This:

fi you can raed tihs, you have a sgtrane mind too. I cdnuolt blveiee that I aulaclty uesdnatnrd what I was rdanieg. The phaonmneal pweor of the human mind, aoccdrig to a rscheearch at Cmabrigde Uinervtisy, it dseno't mtaetr in what oerdr the ltteres in a word are, the only iproamtnt thing is that the frsit and lsat ltteer be in the rghit pclae. The rset can be a taotl mses and you can still raed it whotuit a pboerlm. This is bcuseae the human mind deos not raed ervey lteter by istlef, but the word as a wlohe. Azanmig huh? Yaeh and I awlyas tghuhot slpeling was ipmorantt!

MORE FUN FACTS

The reason why the wedding ring is placed on the fourth finger of your left hand is that it's the only finger that has a vein connecting directly to your heart.

People say "Bless You" when you sneeze, because when you sneeze, your heart stops for a mili-second.

The average woman will spend one year of her life trying to decide what to wear!

If you are willing to sit in bed for 87 days for research on the effects of zero gravity on your body, NASA will pay you $15,000. (wtffunfact.com)

To play "Happy Birthday" on your phone, dial:

112163 112196 11#9632 969363

Brain Foods: Answers

FUN WITH NUMBERS:

Answer = 8!

Your number is 5!

JUST FOR FUN:

What building has the most stories? (A Library!)

What can be swallowed, but can also swallow you?
(Water!)

What can clap without any hands? (Thunder!)

A woman has seven children. Half of them are boys. How
is this possible? (They are all boys!)

The 22nd and 24th presidents of the U.S. had the same
parents but were not brothers. How can this be possible?
(They were the same man.)

What has no weight, but is heavy enough to sink a ship? (A
hole.)

My friend can shave over 10 times a day but still has a full beard. How can this be possible? (He is the barber.)

The mayor of the city has a brother. His name is John. John says he doesn't have a brother. How can this be possible? (The mayor is a woman.)

Can you find the the mistake 1 2 3 4 5 6 7 8 9 10? (The word *the* appears twice.)

Chapter Thirteen: Success Stories

Diane Brown
(Morrilton, AR)

I don't remember being teased, or even feeling overweight during my elementary school days. My first thoughts of actually feeling "fat" (I'll never forget that feeling) were when I begin attending junior high school, 7th grade.

What happened to the 6th or even the 5th grades? I don't know.

In my opinion, my "HIPS" were gigantic! I was always pulling my shirts and t-shirts down over those "monstrous hips." Now, I know this was my first introduction to *"Overweight."*

No, I didn't do anything about my weight during those younger years. However, as an adult and having been married and given birth to three children, I typically tried to keep my weight between 150-163 lbs. and my dress size between a 12-14. Sometimes, I'd go as high as 16. Oddly enough, the heavier I was, the more I learned to "love" my "HIPS!" They gave me the appearance of a smaller waistline!

This was especially true for the size 16 because then "HIPS" became my "best friend."

I got involved with aerobic classes and focused on eating *somewhat* healthy.

Then, "life" happened. I got divorced.

Of course, divorce doesn't just happen; sometimes the *process* can take years before you actually get there. During those *process* years, I went from weighing 150 pounds to weighing 175.

When I began buying clothes that were a size 20, THAT was MY rock bottom, my turn-around! Something clicked inside me. I told myself, "This is it! You must get out of this place that you have gotten yourself."

My body (standing only 5'2") was in pain. Bending was miserable. Clothes looked horrible on me, but the thing that bothered me the most was my lack of self-esteem. I was not happy; however, for my small children, I had to wear a "happy face."

In order for me to win this 'battle of the bulge,' I knew there were three things I was going to need:

- **Motivation**: Get and stay focused!
- **Will-Power**: Make a plan and put it into action (attack it)!
- **Perseverance**: Keep going no matter how hard it seemed!

I Prayed! And God did it!

It was a Monday morning. I woke up on "GO!" I went radical!

I began working out 3-times a day (morning, noon, and before I went to bed at night). I ate only healthy foods, vegetables, grilled or baked meats and drank plenty of water. Within the first three months, I lost 30 pounds! I had already reached my first goal, which was to get back to my comfort size.

I realized that my battle words (*motivation, will-power,* and *perseverance*) were still burning strong! So, I too stayed the race - literally. By this time, I was running 3-5 miles, 5-6 days a week. In two months, I lost 20 more pounds.

I was now healthy! I felt great! My self-esteem returned, and now, I was happy with no more fake "happy faces!"

That's my story. It would be the first of my many "weight loss" journeys.

I'm still very conscious of my weight, so I'll always be a "loser" because I choose to be healthy, not just body wise, but in my soul and mind too.

Not being at "my" comfortable weight affected all of those areas.

This next thing I'm about to say is of the utmost importance.

To all who read my story, just know that each individual's 'comfort place' can be different.

And that's OK!

Questions to consider:

- Do you know your comfort place?
- What triggered your weight gain?
- Are you happy and healthy?

_____

_____

_____

_____

_____

Iris M. Williams

(Little Rock, AR)

I think if people saw pictures of me before the age of six (incredibly skinny) and pictures of me ten years ago (incredibly fat), they wouldn't recognize me. I look at those pictures and don't recognize me!

Now that I know what I know (weight gain is a symptom of pain), I realize that the death of my father (pain) and unhealthy relationships (more pain) were the catalyst for my weight gain. Of course, the more weight I gained, the more miserable I became.

Others would tell me that I was 'pretty' and that I wasn't fat, but I always felt trapped in a body that didn't serve me. Don't get me wrong; my outside matched my inside – I was miserable. However, I didn't want to be. I wanted to be happy, free, and most of all I wanted to be honest.

When you are not happy, you tend to feel that you have to pretend to be happy so others can feel comfortable around you. After so many years of being a liar, I decided I wanted to be a loser!

I needed new pants. The size 24 that I had at home were now too tight. As I walked around the store disgusted at myself and the limited selection, I knew I had to do something.

Of course, I wanted quick results!

I ordered this diet plan off the television and was determined to give it a try. It was not my first attempt; however, I think this one worked because I was tired. I was tired of my life and the way I "wasn't" living it. My job was threatening to base our insurance premiums on weight and health. I knew that would include me. At the screening, I was told that I was borderline diabetic, that my blood pressure was high, and that it needed to be monitored. I have never like taking medicines, so all of this was the perfect storm. It was time to do something.

The diet I chose boiled down to me eating six times a day. I rarely ate more than twice a day. It also meant baked chicken and grapefruit. I usually ate red meat daily and rarely ate fruit or vegetables unless they were covered in some kind of heavy sauce. The first day of the diet, I cried. I was crying because I had let myself go. I checked the list of people I cared for and realized I wasn't listed.

The diet worked. I lost about twenty pounds and felt great.

That 'kick start' motivated me to keep going.

I joined Weight Watchers and decided I wanted to make 'lifestyle' changes. Slowly, I replaced unhealthy foods and habits with ones that were not only healthier, but ones that I knew would become a permanent part of my diet and life.

Weight is not something that you focus on for a time just to stop. Like most things, it requires constant attention. These days, I eat (or have a meal replacement shake) regularly. I'm a size 16, and that seems to feel comfortable to me. I like how I look in my clothes, and most importantly, I love how I feel inside. Finally, my insides are matching my outsides!

I recognize that I'll be a *loser* for the rest of my life.

I'm ok with that.

Questions to consider:

- Do your insides match your outsides?
- Who in your life tells you the truth?
- Why do you think diets fail?

Troy Crittenden
(Atlanta, Georgia)

My wake-up call began in March 2015, then at the age of 36, (215pounds, height 5'6) during my company's "Employee Wellness Check" I was found to have dangerously high blood pressure numbers. I was advised to see my family doctor ASAP. I signed on to participate in my first 5k walk/run with my co-workers. During the walk, I had a lot of time to reflect on my health, and well-being and if I would even live to see age 40. Towards the last stretch of the race, I had *decided to make a decision.*

After I completed the 5k, I went to the grocery store, stocked up on frozen veggies, bottled water, and chicken breast. I told myself, I'm going see what eating right and working out does and feels like. By the end of 3 weeks, I was 11 pounds lighter; by 6 weeks I was 18 pounds lighter. By 15 weeks, my weight loss was very noticeable by my co-workers, I not only had lost weight, but I also looked 10 years younger, my blood pressure amazingly went back to normal.

It's now 2018, and I work out six days a week. I continue a healthy eating regimen, allow myself one cheat "meal" (not cheat day) on the weekends, and as a result, I lost a total of 52 pounds in 4-1/2 months. I'm now maintaining at 163 pounds.

I FEEL GREAT AND SO CAN YOU!

Questions to consider:

- Do you know your numbers?
- Have you thought about your health goals?
- Do you have a plan?

_____

_____

_____

_____

_____

Chapter Fourteen: Size, Serving, Protein & Emotion

Portion Size Guide

Do you know how a 3oz serving of meat looks? 2tbsp of oil, 1 cup pasta, or you aware that there or some foods that have unlimited portions!

Well, check this out!

3 ounces of meat = equivalent to a *deck of cards*

1c pasta = Tennis ball size

¼c fruit = light bulb size

½c dried fruit = golf ball size

1oz cheese = 1 domino size

3oz fish = checkbook size

1 tsp oil = size of 1 dice

½c rice = cupcake wrapper size

1c cereal = size of a fist

1 baked potato = computer mouse size

2tbsp peanut butter = size of a golf ball

1 cookie = top of a soda can size

½c ice cream = cupcake wrapper size

1oz nuts = sm. Dixie cup

2tbsp salad dressing = shot glass size

Serving of Dark chocolate = dental floss box size

½c pretzels, crackers = 1 cupped hand (palm)

Daily Recommendation from Food Group & Its Serving *(Thrivemarket.com)*

FRUIT GROUP:

4 half cup servings of fruit= ½ apple, ½ lg orange, ½ lg banana, 4 lg strawberries, ¼c dried fruit or 16 seedless grapes.

VEGETABLE GROUP:

3 1 cup servings= 1 lg tomato, 1med. baked sweet potato, 1 heaping handful of most veggies, 2 med. whole carrots, or 2c raw greens (spinach, kale, romaine, watercress, escarole)

GRAINS:

6-8 one oz servings = 1 reg. slice of bread, ½c cooked oatmeal, ½c cooked pasta or rice, 7 square or round crackers, or 3 cups popcorn (plain)

PROTEIN: 2 ½ - 3 two-ounce servings per day = ½ - ¾ can of tuna, 2 eggs, ½c cooked beans, small 2oz steak or 24 almonds (Dixie cup size).

High Protein Vegetables You Need to Start Eating Today!
(healthy-holistic-living.com and ncbi.nlm.nih.gov)

I bet you thought I'd forgotten. There are some unlimited food portions! Yes, you can indulge - *VEGETABLES!* But, get to know your vegetables! For you who didn't know there are starchy vegetables, winter squash, corn, and lima beans are just a few).

Below, I have listed a few of the High Protein Veggies (who knew, besides vegetarians) there was such a thing as *"Protein Vegetables."*

Watercress- Has been shown to offer antioxidant protection. It also contains phenolic compounds that may help prevent cancer (pgs.2-6).

Alfalfa Sprouts- have been shown to decrease inflammation, reduce symptoms of menopause, and help treat and prevent osteoporosis. ref: ncbi.nlm.nih.gov

Spinach- Regularly consuming spinach has been linked to as much as a 44% lower risk of breast cancer (pg.20). ncbi.nlm.nih.gov

Chinese Cabbage or Bok Choy- Chinese cabbage is used in many Asian recipes, such as stir-fries, kimchi, soups, and spring rolls.

Asparagus- is thought to have anti-inflammatory and anticancer properties (pg.28). ncbi.nlm.nih.gov

Mustard Greens- Test study shows that steamed mustard greens may help reduce cholesterol levels (pg.33).

Broccoli- can help improve liver health (pg.40)!

Collard Greens- one study reported that people who eat cruciferous vegetables like collard greens are less likely to be diagnosed with breast cancer (pg.25).

Brussels Sprouts- A study in animals showed that brussels sprouts could promote the growth and health of intestinal bacteria and stimulate the production of short-chain fatty acids in the gut (pg.45).

Last, but not least, cauliflower contains a high amount of a compound called, *sinigrin.* This is thought to have anticancer, antioxidant, and anti-inflammatory properties (pgs.38,47,48).

Food Aids for Emotions
(Everyday Health)

There are eight foods that help fight depression. Your diet may provide a complementary or alternative depression treatment. Learn foods that may help depression. Turkey has a high level of a chemical called, tryptophan.

1. Walnuts are rich in omega3.
2. Fatty Fish has brain-boosting properties.
3. Low-fat dairy has 2 powerhouse nutrients, calcium and Vitamin D.
4. Whole Grains help the body release *serotonin*.
5. Green Tea has an amino acid known as, *theanine,* found in tea leaves that provides an anti-stress relaxation benefit to tea drinkers.
6. Tumeric is a bold spice found in many Indian and Asian curry dishes which is a great way to *boost your mood.*
7. Dark Chocolate helps to release *serotonin* and relaxes the blood vessels of the cardiovascular system. But because dark chocolate is so calorie dense, its suggested to eat just 1 small piece.

Get Real

At the end of the day, the opinion that matters is yours. If you're sick of living a lie or being unsatisfied, or craving change, the only person who can address those feelings and thoughts is you. Be mindful about what you eat.

Here are a few things to consider:

*Need the motivation to lose weight, try eating in front of a mirror naked.

*What you eat in private, you wear in public.

*The first step to getting anywhere is deciding you're not willing to stay where you are.

*Watch your habits, not your weight.

*The hard part isn't getting your body in shape. The hard part is getting your mind in shape.

*Losing weight is hard; being fat is hard. *PICK YOUR HARD*.

*You are not hungry; you are bored. Drink some water and learn *the difference.*

*Healthy Self = *Heal thy Self*

*I'm not trying to look perfect...I just want to feel better, look great, know I'm healthy and be able to *ROCK* any outfit I choose!

*Strong is the new beautiful.

*When I lost all of my *Excuses*, I found all of my *Results!*

*Don't expect to see a change, if you don't make one.

*It's just a hill, get over it.

*If you're tired of starting over, stop giving up.

*Make it happen, shock everyone!

*If I quit now, I will soon be back to where I started, and when I started, I desperately wished to be where I am now.

*Fat lasts longer than flavor

*Fitness is about being better than you use to be.

*No matter how slowly you go, you are still lapping everybody on the couch.

*Fitness is 100% *Mental*! Your body won't go where your mind doesn't push it.

*Do not *reward* yourself with food...you're not a dog.

*Don't dig your grave with your own knife and fork.

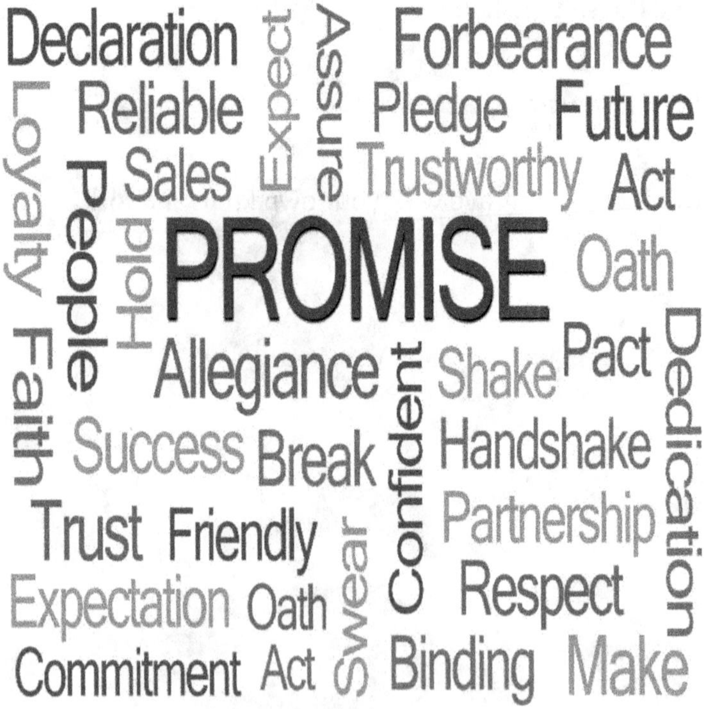
PROMISE
Declaration
Expect
Assure
Forbearance
Loyalty
Reliable
Pledge
Future
People
Sales
Trustworthy
Act
Hold
Oath
Faith
Allegiance
Confident
Shake
Pact
Dedication
Success
Break
Handshake
Trust
Friendly
Partnership
Swear
Expectation
Oath
Respect
Commitment
Act
Binding
Make

Contract for Change

Dear Body,

I'm sorry I've treated you this way, feeding you the wrong foods, and not taking care of you. I promise to do better and get you back to the best shape and fitness level you can be; we can do it!

Sincerely,

Me

Contract For Change

The "Loser"!

_____

My Path to Wellness Begins Here …

Date:

Click here to enter text.

This contract is simply a reminder for myself that dieting is not just about how I look, but also about how I feel. I understand that change begins with me. I will identify motivators and well as stressors. I will be mindful of what I eat as well as the amount of activity and/or movement that I incorporate in my daily living.

Personal Goal:

_____

_____

Motivating Factors:

_____

_____

Changes Needed To Reach Goal:

_____

_____

Plan For Making Changes:

_____

_____

I'm A Loser by Diane Brown

Start Date:

_____

Assessment Plan:

_____

_____

Support System (If I Need Help):

Name	Phone	Email

Target Date To Reach Goal:

_____

Reward(s) For Achieving Goal:

_____

_____

The Witness!   The "Loser"!

By: _____   By: _____
Name: Name:
Title: Title:

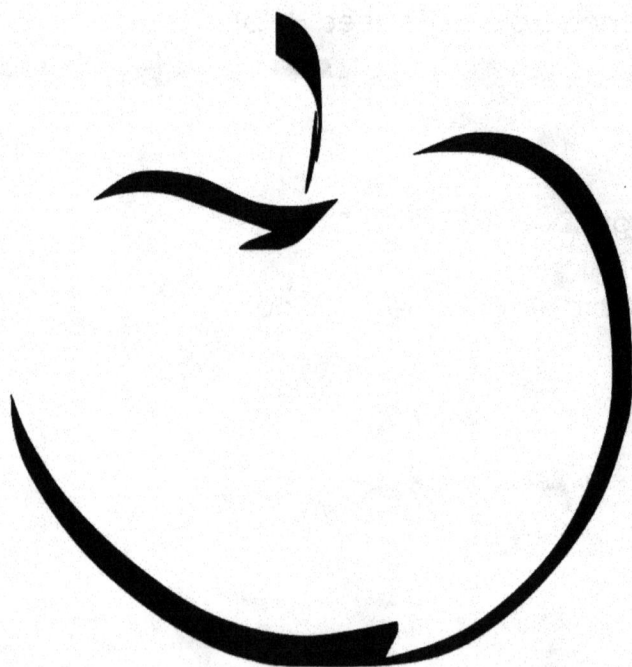

About the Author

Author Diane Brown is a 'lifetime loser' and wants you to be one too. The author has successfully managed her weight for years. She once thought that there would come a time when she wouldn't have to worry about weight, but one day she noticed that her 90-year-young mother was still dieting!

That's when it hit her that healthy living and eating were a lifestyle.

"I have accepted the reality that 'diet' is a lifestyle. Therefore, the journey doesn't end! The desire to look and feel your best should continue. I've now become a member of the "Losers Club," and I want YOU to join me."

You may contact the author via

Email: Lose2Win59@hotmail.com

Facebook: Diane Brown   Lose2Win

Phone (messages only): 501-354-4205

Butterfly Typeface Publishing

Books to intelligently entertain
the discriminating reader!

Contact us for all your

publishing & writing needs!

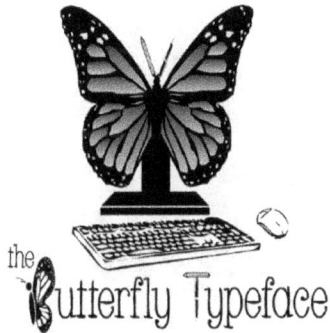

the Butterfly Typeface

Iris M Williams

PO Box 56193

Little Rock AR 72215www.butterflytypeface.com

www.ingramcontent.com/pod-product-compliance
Lightning Source LLC
Chambersburg PA
CBHW072125270326
41931CB00010B/1678